RACIAL PRESCRIPTIONS

Racial Prescriptions

Pharmaceuticals, Difference, and the Politics of Life

JONATHAN XAVIER INDA
University of Illinois, Urbana-Champaign, USA

Routledge
Taylor & Francis Group
LONDON AND NEW YORK

First published 2014 by Routledge

2 Park Square, Milton Park, Abingdon, Oxon OX14 4RN
711 Third Avenue, New York, NY 10017, USA

Routledge is an imprint of the Taylor & Francis Group, an informa business

First issued in paperback 2016

British Library Cataloguing in Publication Data
A catalogue record for this book is available from the British Library

The Library of Congress has cataloged the printed edition as follows:
Inda, Jonathan Xavier.
Racial prescriptions : pharmaceuticals, difference, and the politics of life / by Jonathan Xavier Inda.
pages cm
Includes bibliographical references and index.

ISBN 978-1-4094-4498-5 (hbk)
ISBN 978-1-138-69569-6 (pbk)

1. Discrimination in medical care. 2. Health services accessibility. 3. Minorities--Medical care. 4. Social medicine. I. Title.

RA563.M56I53 2014
362.1089--dc23

2014012543

Contents

Acknowledgments *vii*

1 Racial Politics of Life 1

2 The Making of BiDil 23

3 Biosocial Citizenship 39

4 Enlightened Geneticization of Race 57

5 Racial Vital Value 75

6 Neoliberalization of Life 93

Bibliography *111*
Index *133*

Acknowledgments

This book could not have been completed without the aid, support, and feedback of numerous friends and colleagues. Special thanks go to Monica Casper, Laura Cremonesi, Paisley Currah, Orazio Irrera, Daniele Lorenzini, Rebecca Martinez, Anne Pollock, Amit Prasad, Srirupa Prasad, Martina Tazzioli, and the anonymous reviewers at Ashgate. They all provided incisive critiques and commentary that greatly enhanced the book.

I also thank audiences at the various institutions and conferences where I presented portions of the book: the Department of Women's and Gender Studies at the University of Missouri; the Unit for Criticism and Interpretive Theory's "Bios: Life, Death, Politics" Conference at the University of Illinois, Urbana-Champaign; the American Sociological Association's 2010 Annual Meeting; and the BIOS Centre's "Vital Politics III" Conference at the London School of Economics.

Many thanks go to the faculty and staff of the Department of Latina/ Latino Studies at the University of Illinois at Urbana-Champaign—Adrian Burgos, Lisa Cacho, Jorge Chapa, Laura Castañeda, David Coyoca, Edna Viruell-Fuentes, Mireya Loza, Alejandro Lugo, Isabel Molina, Alicia P. Rodriguez, Richard T. Rodriguez, Rolando Romero, Gilberto Rosas, and Sandra Ruiz—for providing a supportive and invigorating environment in which to carry out my work.

I must express my gratitude to Neil Jordan at Ashgate for his enthusiastic support of the project, to Stephanie Ceman at the University of Illinois for teaching me about medical genetics, and to Alice Morrow Rowan for her wonderful editing work.

For financial assistance, I am grateful to the College of Liberal Arts and Sciences at the University of Illinois. A Faculty Study in a Second Discipline award gave me time off from teaching to study genetics. I must also thank the Illinois Campus Research Board; through their Humanities Released Time program I was given a semester off to work on the book.

Finally, I wish to thank my wife, Julie, and my daughter, Sofia, for their love and support. Words can barely begin to express how much they mean to me and how much joy they bring to my life. This book is dedicated to them.

Parts of this book draw on previously published work. Chapter 1 appeared in modified form as "For blacks only: farmaci, genetica e politica razziale della vita," *Materiali Foucaultiani*, 1[2] (2012), 107–35. A much different version of Chapter 3 was published as "Materializing hope: racial pharmaceuticals, suffering bodies, and biological citizenship," in *Corpus: An Interdisciplinary Reader on Bodies and Knowledge*, edited by M. Casper and P. Currah (New York: Palgrave Macmillan, 2011), 61–80. Finally, Chapter 6 is informed by the theorization of post-social government in *Targeting Immigrants: Government, Technology, and Ethics* (Malden, MA: Wiley-Blackwell, 2006).

Chapter 1
Racial Politics of Life

On June 16, 2005, the Cardiovascular and Renal Drugs Advisory Committee of the US Food and Drug Administration (FDA) held a daylong meeting to discuss a new drug application for BiDil (US FDA 2005a). The drug was being considered for approval to treat African Americans suffering from congestive heart failure, a condition in which the heart is unable to pump sufficient blood to the body's other organs. In addition to the committee members, gathered together were FDA consultants, representatives of NitroMed (the maker of BiDil), and a number of other guests, from medical scientists and academics to heart failure sufferers and spokespeople for various African American and minority civil rights, professional, and political organizations.

Following a series of speakers from NitroMed, most of whom addressed the scientific evidence pointing to BiDil's efficacy, the committee opened the floor for comments from the public. One individual who spoke was Debra Lee, a 48-year-old African American woman with heart failure. She was there to tell her story. "In 1999," she stated, "I had a heart attack. There was blockage in my heart. A stent was inserted. In early 2003 I noticed a change in my health—coughing continuously; being visibly short of breath; walking short distances tired me out; waking up in the middle of the night; sleeping in a chair because I felt as if I would suffocate if I laid down" (Lee 2005: 218). Doctors tested Lee for various conditions, and in August 2003 she was diagnosed with congestive heart failure.

Later that year, Lee was offered a chance to participate in the African American Heart Failure Trial (A-HeFT), a clinical trial cosponsored by NitroMed and the Association of Black Cardiologists (ABC) to test BiDil in self-identified black patients. She quickly said yes. How was Lee feeling at the time of her testimony? "I feel fabulous," she narrated. "No more shortness of breath; I am able to walk and exercise without resting; I can sleep in my bed at night; I am working more hours at the Indianapolis Museum of Art; I have more energy" (2005: 219). And to what did she attribute this turnaround? "It is my strong faith in God," Lee said, "and a little pill called BiDil. I believe this pill is helping my heart to pump stronger. ... In my opinion, this pill has changed so many things for me, given me a new lease on life. ... I believe I have another 40 years or so to live my life to its fullest" (2005: 219–20).

The story that Debra Lee narrated is at once about a suffering body and about a body of hope. It is about the pain that comes with a debilitating, chronic, and fatal condition such as heart failure: the shortness of breath, the persistent coughing, the fatigue, the increased heart rate—and the list goes on. It is also about the expectation that BiDil will not only prolong life but also improve the quality of one's existence. This mobilization of suffering and hope was not unique to Lee's story. The imagery appeared time and again in other testimonies delivered during the open public hearing (US FDA 2005a). A case in point is Congresswoman Donna Christensen. Speaking as chair of the Congressional Black Caucus Health Braintrust, she began her testimony by painting a portrait of black suffering, underscoring the health disparities that befall this population. "Every day," she stated, "more than 200 African Americans die from premature causes. The leading cause of those deaths is heart disease, which we suffer more disproportionately from than any other racial or ethnic group. Heart failure among African Americans is expected to increase from 725,000 to 900,000 in the next five years, and 50 percent of those patients survive less than five years after diagnosis" (Christensen 2005: 204). In this context, Congresswoman Christensen saw BiDil as an opportunity to substantially reduce health inequities. Highlighting data from A-HeFT, she noted that the drug reduced the mortality of trial participants by 43 percent, decreased their rates of hospitalization from heart failure by one-third, and generally improved their quality of life. For Congresswoman Christensen, BiDil was thoroughly imbued with hope and the prospect of saving black lives. As she put it, "BiDil can save thousands of lives and reduce untold suffering for African American heart failure patients and their families" (2005: 209).

Significantly, not everyone at the public forum regarded BiDil with a high degree of optimism. Although all of the speakers agreed that the drug should be approved, there were some who argued that to restrict its use to just African Americans and not make it available to the general population was highly problematic. Among the critics was Shomarka Keita, an anthropologist affiliated with the Smithsonian Institution and the National Human Genome Center at Howard University. His main concern, one shared by others, was that the case for BiDil seemed to be based on the idea that African Americans have a specific biological and presumably genetic profile that makes the drug more effective in them than in European Americans. This reasoning implies that African Americans constitute a discrete biological-genetic grouping. According to Keita, however, such is simply not the case. As he put it, "The African American group does not consist of uniform individuals who are biologically the same, due to genealogical uniformity, or even environmental insult" (Keita 2005: 222). Rather, this population is strictly a social entity. The implications of this view for how BiDil should be indicated are significant. As Keita further noted, "Medications work at the levels of pathophysiology, clinical phenotypes and individuals and not on sociodemographic categories, groups or mystical identities" (2005: 222). Thus, to the extent that African Americans are a social group and not a genetic one, there is no reason to believe that BiDil would work on all members of this population and not at all on other populations. Drugs just do not work on the basis of socially designated racial and ethnic categories; instead, their efficacy is linked to specific genotypes that are shared across populations. Ultimately, Keita recommended that BiDil should not be indicated for just African Americans and suggested the need to identify "the specific pathophysiology, clinical phenotype on which the components of BiDil work" and to treat "the susceptible clinical phenotype in any and all individuals who have it irrespective of origin" (2005: 222–3). Left unsaid in all this, but certainly a subtext, was a strong concern regarding the biologization of race. Given the United States' historical experience with racial science, in which some groups have been classified as biologically inferior and others as superior, to geneticize African Americans and designate BiDil as a racial drug was potentially to open the door to ethnic stereotyping, discrimination, and marginalization.

At the end of the day, the Cardiovascular and Renal Drugs Advisory Committee, citing among other things the "disproportionate burdens of heart failure in blacks" and the need to develop effective treatment in this population "in light of health disparities," recommended the approval of BiDil for African Americans (Nissen 2005: 2046). Saving African American lives seemed to trump any concerns with the problems of biologizing race. A week later, on June 23, the FDA, following the committee's recommendation, approved the drug "for the treatment of heart failure in self-identified black patients" (US FDA 2005b). BiDil thus became the first drug endorsed by the FDA for a specific racial group (Meadows 2005).

In this book, I explore the contemporary politics of race and pharmaceuticals through the prism of BiDil. Drawing on Michel Foucault's work on biopower (discussed in the next section), I specifically look at how BiDil is implicated in what could be called a *racial politics of life*. This is a politics that takes as its object the biological vitality of the racial body. In the contemporary United States, matters of life and health have undoubtedly become key political concerns (Ong 2006, Rose 2007). Indeed, fostering the vitality of the living body—through practices ranging from basic primary care to high-tech medicine and pharmaceuticals—has developed into a central objective of political and other authorities. Important to this politics of vitality is the desire to overcome racial disparities in health. From heart disease and diabetes to cancer and asthma, the populations most afflicted by a range of illnesses are racialized minorities (African Americans, Latinos, Native Americans, and so forth). The solutions generally proposed to the problem of racial health disparities have been social and environmental (for example, better access to health care and improved living conditions), but in the wake of the mapping of the human genome, genetic thinking has come to have considerable influence on how such inequalities are problematized. Increasingly, a strongly held belief among scientists, medical researchers, and politicians is that notable differences exist between racial groups at the genomic level and that these differences are medically significant (Risch et al. 2002). They thus contend that racial classification is necessary in order to target those diseases that most affect disadvantaged racial minorities and to remedy the underrepresentation of these populations in medical research, drug development, and access to health care. The hope is that genetically-based medicine will play a central role in ameliorating race-based health inequalities. Pharmaceuticals targeted at specific racial groups are key to this politics of life. The personalization of therapeutics promises to bring the benefits of modern medicine to often socially excluded populations.

The book pays particular attention to three dimensions of the vital politics of racialized pharmaceuticals. First, it deals with how matters of health, disease, and bodily suffering have come to be linked with questions of rights and citizenship. It is concerned, that is, with how individuals and populations nowadays often make claims on—and are recognized by—political, medical, and other authorities in terms of "their 'vital' rights as citizens" (Rose and Novas 2005: 441). Medications intended specifically for minority populations are, on some level, precisely about vital rights. They are about entitlement to health care, hoping for cures, and aiding suffering bodies.

Second, the book explores the problem of race and biology. Although racialized pharmaceuticals are ostensibly about fostering the vital forces of the biological body, their politics of life also raises thorny questions about the biologization of race. Some social scientists and other scholars have questioned how medicine can legitimately employ the notion of race when it has time and again been deemed scientifically tenuous (Lee, Mountain, and Koenig 2001, Fujimura, Duster, and Rajagopalan 2008, Whitmarsh and Jones 2010). Drawing on a wealth of population genetics research, they conclude that distinct races do not exist and that there is simply no biological justification for so-called racial groups. At issue for these critics is the likelihood that looking for health equity through the biological lens of race will lead to the naturalization of health disparities, permitting biological explanations to overshadow social, economic, and ecological understandings of disease (Fullwiley 2007). A key concern of the book is to interrogate the ways in which race has been biologized through the making of pharmaceuticals, and the implications of this biologization.

Third, the book examines the capitalization of racial life. By and large, the production of health and vitality in the United States has come to be linked closely to the generation of wealth (Franklin 2000, Rose 2007). Indeed, biomedicine and the life sciences in general are nowadays highly subject to the demands of capitalization, such that commercial considerations (that is, shareholder demands and profit obligations) heavily shape the medical problems they seek to address. Pharmaceutical companies have played an important role in this capitalization of life. Through the production of pharmaceuticals, they aim not only to boost the vitality of the living but also, and perhaps more importantly, to generate economic value. In this context, the racial body has emerged as a potentially valuable biocommodity (Abu El-Haj 2007). Race-based pharmaceuticals hold out the promise of yielding significant economic profit.

Overall, the book explores the politics of dealing with health disparities by targeting pharmaceuticals at specific racial groups on the basis of the idea that they are genetically different. It suggests that although drugs such as BiDil might help save African American lives, and bring a measure of hope to a community that historically has been denied access to the benefits of modern medicine, we need to be mindful not to obscure the social significance of race and not to reduce health disparities to health differences grounded simply in biology and genetics (Kahn 2005). In neglecting the social, there is a danger that medical and societal inequities will simply intensify with race-based medicine. We also need to be wary of how race can be misused to create market opportunities. Indeed, by treating race as a valuable biocommodity, there is always the possibility that making profits might trump saving lives.

Foucault on Biopower

Intellectually, this book takes Michel Foucault's work on biopower as its point of departure.[1] In the final chapter of *The History of Sexuality* (1980), Foucault notes that for a long time one of the basic prerogatives of sovereign power was the right to decide life and death. For instance, if an external enemy sought to overthrow the sovereign, the latter could justly wage war, requiring his subjects to fight in defense of the state. So, without directly causing his subjects' deaths, the sovereign was sanctioned to risk their lives, thus exercising an indirect power of life and death over them. If, however, someone hazarded to rebel against the sovereign and violate his laws, the sovereign could exert a direct power over the transgressor's life, such that the latter could be put to death. The right to life and death was thus somewhat asymmetrical, weighted on the side of death. As Foucault puts it, "The sovereign exercised his right to life only by exercising his right to kill, or by refraining from killing; he evidenced his power over life only through the death he was capable of requiring. The right which was formulated as the

1 This book is also in dialogue with and seeks to contribute to the important body of literature that has developed around the theme of race, genetics, science, and medicine. Important works include Reardon 2005, Epstein 2007, Koenig, Lee, and Richardson 2008, Whitmarsh 2008, Metzl 2009, Whitmarsh and Jones 2010, Fullwiley 2011, Montoya 2011, Morning 2011, Roberts 2011a, 2011b, Bliss 2012, Pollock 2012, Wailoo, Nelson, and Lee 2012, Happe 2013, Hartigan 2013 and Kahn 2013.

'power of life and death' was in reality the right to *take* life or *let* live" (1980: 136). Ultimately, sovereign power functioned mainly as a mechanism of deduction—as a means to appropriate a portion of the wealth, labor, services, and blood of the sovereign's subjects. As such, it was fundamentally a right of seizure that culminated in the license to take hold of life in order to subdue it.

This power of appropriation or deduction, Foucault suggests, is no longer the principal form of political power in the West. Since the seventeenth century, the mechanisms of power have undergone a radical transformation. Power now generally works to organize, control, reinforce, monitor, incite, and optimize the energies of individual and collective life. It is not focused on impeding or destroying life but on generating it, making it grow, and ordering it. Thus, in contrast to a power organized around a sovereign, modern power does not "deal simply with legal subjects over whom the ultimate dominion [is] death, but with living beings" (1980: 142–3). Indeed, Foucault suggests that power's supreme function is no longer to kill but to invest thoroughly in life. It is over life that modern political power establishes its hold and on which it seeks to have a positive influence. The name that Foucault gives to this power over life is *biopower*. It essentially designates "what brought life and its mechanisms into the realm of explicit calculations and made knowledge-power an agent of transformation of human life" (1980: 143).

Biopower, according to Foucault (1980: 139), has assumed two basic forms in the West. One form, which he calls a *biopolitics of the population*, or simply *biopolitics*, is concerned with population at "the level of its aggregate effects" (2000: 219). Here biopower takes as its target the population regarded as a species body: "the body imbued with the mechanics of life and serving as the basis of the biological processes: propagation, births and mortality, the level of health, life expectancy and longevity, with all the conditions that can cause these to vary" (1980: 139). Put otherwise, biopolitics attends to the biological processes of the collective social body. It is concerned with regulating the phenomena that typify groups of living human beings: reproduction and human sexuality, the size and quality of the population, health and illness, living and working conditions, birth and death, and the like. The goal of biopolitics is to optimize the life of the population as a whole. The second form, which Foucault calls an *anatamo-politics of the human body*, or simply *discipline*, "implies the management of population in its depths and its details" (2000: 219). Here biopower centers not on the population as a whole but on the individual bodies that compose it. Indeed, the target of discipline is not the collective but the individual human body—taken as an object to be manipulated. The goal of discipline is to produce human beings whose bodies are at once useful and docile. It is to optimize the life of the body: to augment its capabilities, extort its forces, and increase its utility and docility. Biopower thus amounts to nothing less than the taking charge of life by political power. It points to how political and other authorities have assigned themselves the duty of administering bodies and managing collective life.

Significantly, although Foucault argues that the governing of bodies and the calculated management of life has supplanted the old power of death that typified sovereign power, this does not mean that the right of death has altogether disappeared. Rather, it has experienced a shift, or at least "a tendency to align itself with the exigencies of a life-administering power and to define itself accordingly" (1980: 136). Put otherwise, the awesome power of death "now represents itself as the counterpart of a power that exerts a positive influence on life, that endeavors to administer, optimize, and multiply it, subjecting it to precise controls and comprehensive regulations" (1980: 137). Yet, as Foucault notes, modern wars are bloodier than ever, and never before have regimes subjected their own populations to such wanton holocausts (Nazi Germany, for example). But if genocide is an effect of modern power, this is not by virtue of the restitution of the sovereign right to kill, but because power is located and practiced at the level of life. Indeed, wars are no longer conducted in the name of the sovereign. They are waged in defense of collective existence. It is in order to nurture life—the life of the population—that life can be disallowed. As Foucault puts it, "entire populations are mobilized for the purpose of wholesale slaughter in the name of life necessity. ... It is as managers of life and survival, of bodies and the race, that so many regimes have been able to wage so many wars, causing so many men to be killed" (1980: 139).

Foucault further elucidates this underside of biopower in the last lecture of *Society Must Be Defended* (2003). There he asks, because biopower's "objective is to make live, how can it let die? How can the power of death, the function of death, be exercised in a political system centered upon biopower?" (2003: 254). His answer is *racism.* Within a regime of power aimed at fostering life, Foucault notes, racism is the necessary precondition that makes killing permissible. It essentially introduces "a break into the domain of life that is under power's control: the break between what must live and what must die" (2003: 254). Racism works to introduce this break in two ways. First, it takes the biological continuum of the human species and divides it up into races, designating certain ones as good and others as inferior. Second, it sets up a relation between one's life and the death of others such that the more one kills and permits others to die, the more one will live. This relationship, according to Foucault, is one of war. The enemies that have to be eliminated, however, are not adversaries in a political sense. Rather, they are biological foes—internal and external threats to the species or population. The idea here is that the death of the other, the death of the bad or inferior race, will make life in general more healthy and pure. This death does not have to be direct death or the literal act of putting to death. It could also be indirect death: the act of exposing to death, of multiplying for some the risk of death, or simply political death, expulsion, rejection, or exclusion. In any case, when life becomes a supreme political value, it appears that the logic of war—that one must be capable of killing in order to keep on living—becomes the predominant principle of power, and fostering the life of the population becomes indistinguishable from the fight against and the necessity of eliminating the biological enemy.

Although death continues to function in the technology of biopower, we are no longer dealing with "the ancient right to *take* life or *let* live." Rather, this right has been "replaced by a power to *foster* life or *disallow* it to the point of death" (1980: 138). This means that although the balance between life and death continues to be asymmetrical, it now falls on the side of life. It is to life that power attends, and life can legitimately be taken only in the name of life itself. For Foucault, this historical transformation in the technology of power from that of sovereignty to that of biopower—from a power operating on the principle of the right to kill to one that generally works to foster life—represents a fundamental revolution in the order of politics. It signifies "nothing less than the entry of life into history, that is, the entry of phenomena peculiar to the life of the human species into the order of knowledge and power, into the sphere of political techniques" (1980: 141–2). It speaks to how biological life has come to be reflected in political existence. Ultimately, according to Foucault, this entry of life into the mechanisms of power signals the advent of the modern. "[W]hat might be called a society's 'threshold of modernity' has been reached," he says, "when the life of the species is wagered on its own political strategies" (1980: 143). Foucault thus proposes that the Aristotelian understanding of man as "a living animal with the additional capacity for a political existence" needs to be amended so that it reads: "modern man is an animal whose politics place his existence as a living being in question" (1980: 143).

The Uses of Biopower

Influenced by Foucault's notion of biopower, scholars have mapped out a broad field of inquiry concerned with the politics of life, that is, with how the vital processes of human existence matter when it comes to politics. Within this broad field, researchers have produced a number of important studies on a range of subjects, including health and disease (Fullwiley 2004, Biehl 2007), pregnancy and reproduction (Weir 2006, Mamo 2007), humanitarianism (Redfield 2005, Fassin 2007), refugees and immigration (Fassin 2001, Inda 2007, Ticktin 2011), colonialism (Stoler 1995, Duncan 2007), the politics of death (Agamben 1998, Mbembe 2003), genetics and genomics (Rabinow 1999, Rose 2007), citizenship (Petryna 2002, Rose and Novas 2005, Ong 2006), war (Reid 2006), and neoliberalism (Collier 2011). The perspective of these studies does not amount to a formal methodology or a unifying theory of biopower.

It is actually a perspective that draws attention to biopower as a heterogeneous field of thought and action—to the multiplicity of authorities, knowledges, strategies, and devices that seek to administer individual and collective life, as well as to the diverse types of selves, persons, agents, or identities arising from the endeavor to manage human vitality. Nonetheless, it is possible to identify two general, and often opposing, orientations in the literature.

On one side, there are those scholars who principally associate biopower with its murderous, exclusionary underside. This side has generally been developed in relation to the war on terror, immigrant and refugee politics, concentration camps and other spaces of detention, and genocide. The most influential expounder of this perspective has no doubt been the Italian philosopher Giorgio Agamben. In *Homo Sacer: Sovereign Power and Bare Life* (1998), Agamben explicitly sets out to rework Foucault's thesis on biopower (Neilson 2006, Mills 2008). He makes two separate but related claims. First, he suggests that biopower and sovereignty are not distinct modalities of power but are actually integrated to such an extent that "the production of a biopolitical body" can be said to be "the original activity of sovereign power" (1998: 6). Put otherwise, the inclusion of biological life in the "political realm constitutes the original—if concealed—nucleus of sovereign power" (1998: 6). Second, Agamben rejects the idea that the historical emergence of biopower signaled Western society's entrance into modernity. Instead, he asserts, power over life has been a part of Western politics from at least the time of classical Greece. This means that biopower and sovereignty have operated concurrently since the founding of Western society. Hence, the hallmark of modernity, according to Agamben, is not the rise of biopower but the coming to light, in an unprecedented way, of the ancient tie uniting power and biological life.

At the center of Agamben's reworking of Foucault are the figures of "bare life" and "the camp."[2] Drawing on Plato and Aristotle, he notes that the ancient Greeks did not have a single term to express what we today mean by "life." Instead, they used two semantically and morphologically distinct words: *zoe* (the simple fact of being alive, common to all living things) and *bios* (the form of living specific to an individual or group). Agamben emphasizes that when Plato and Aristotle theorized about life, they used the term *bios*, because what mattered for them was not brute existence but the way of life proper to human beings. Natural life was in fact excluded from the political life of the *polis*

2 A third figure is *homo sacer*, which Agamben takes from Roman legal history. *Homo sacer* is a being who, because of a grave transgression, is cast outside both the political and sacred domains. As such, a *homo sacer* can be killed by anyone with impunity, but cannot be put to death as part of religious ritual. A *homo sacer*'s demise thus cannot count either as murder or sacrifice. For Agamben, *homo sacer* is a specific embodiment of bare life.

(city-state) and restricted to the sphere of the *oikos* (household). It was thus deemed a subject not worthy of political and ethical contemplation. For Agamben, the exclusion of biological life from the *polis* is rather significant. It actually takes place through a fundamental act of sovereignty. Following the work of Carl Schmitt (1985), Agamben understands sovereign power as the capacity to decide on the exception—to decree an emergency wherein conventional legal and constitutional rules are suspended. In such a state of exception, Agamben suggests, subjects are deprived of constitutional rights, reduced to mere living beings, and exposed to the unconditional power of death. The exclusion of natural life from the sphere of politics amounts to a sovereign act insofar as it is based on a decision as to who is granted status in the *polis* and thus subject to its protections, or who is banned from it and thus exposed to unlimited violation. In this sense, the sovereign's act of exclusion results necessarily in the politicization of life. That is, natural life ends up included in the political domain in the form of exclusion; it is set outside politics but nevertheless implicated in it. Significantly, what gets produced through the sovereign act of in/exclusion is bare life. Bare life is not natural life as such but its politicized form. It can be defined as natural life bereft of political status and hence subject to infinite violation.

Importantly, the originary exclusion of biological life from the *polis*, according to Agamben, finds its ultimate expression in the modern concentration camp. Indeed, for him, the camp represents the state of exception par excellence. "Insofar as its inhabitants were stripped of every political status and wholly reduced to bare life," Agamben notes, "the camp was also the most absolute biopolitical space ever to have been realized, in which power confronts nothing but pure life, without any mediation" (1998: 171). The camp here is a space in which, through an act of sovereignty, the normal juridical order is suspended and human life is degraded to its biological minimum (bare life) and subject to mass annihilation. Thus, to the extent that it actualizes, in an extreme fashion, the suppression of life made possible by the exclusion of *zoe* from the *polis*, the camp superdiscloses the intrinsic logic of Western politics. Agamben does not, however, see the camp simply as an exemplary historical manifestation of sovereign power and the state of exception. For him, the camp is actually "the hidden matrix and *nomos* [organizing principle] of the political space in which we are still living" (1998: 166). Agamben's argument is that, in modern Western society, the state of exception has been generalized to such an extent that it is no longer exceptional but the norm, or as he puts it, "the state of exception comes more and more to the foreground as the fundamental political structure and ultimately begins to become the rule" (1998: 20). This means that rather than just describing a locale, the camp is actually an abstract structure that reveals the general logic of contemporary politics: that all subjects are potentially reducible to bare life.

For Agamben, then, biopower appears to be less about the maintenance of life and more about the production of death (or in/exclusion). Indeed, insofar as he argues that biological life is captured in the political realm through a sovereign act of exclusion, and that the camp represents the "fundamental biopolitical paradigm of the West" (1998: 181), Agamben generally centers on biopower as a kind of *thanatopolitics*—a politics of death. This dark side of biopower is clearly visible not only historically in the concentration camp, but also today in the war on terror, the treatment of refugees, immigrant detention centers, geopolitical border policing, shantytown dwellers, export processing zones, and so forth. In each of these cases, the life of individuals and populations is often stripped of juridical protections and degraded to bare life. That is, human life is reduced to its biological minimum, opened to violence, and rendered potentially disposable.

On the other side of the Foucauldian literature there are those scholars who generally associate biopower with its life-affirming qualities. Their work has generally developed in relation to contemporary biomedicine, biotechnology, and the biosciences. One of the more influential reworkings of the concept of biopower from this angle comes from Paul Rabinow and Nikolas Rose (Rabinow 1998, 1999, 2005, Rose 2001, 2007, Rabinow and Rose 2003, 2006). In their individual and collective work, they have sought to rethink biopower in light of developments in the genetic and biological sciences. Like Foucault, Rabinow and Rose's basic argument is that although the economy of biopower no doubt has its circuits of exclusion and can turn into a murderous politics, it generally operates according to "logics of vitality" (Rabinow and Rose 2006: 211). As they put it, "If biopower sutures together the management of life and the management of death, today 'the dream of power' focuses on the pole of life" (Rabinow and Rose 2003: xxx). Their work is thus principally concerned with exploring projects for making life—that is, schemes that have life rather than death as their end. In particular, they focus on how the growth of the biosciences has given shape to new ways of knowing and intervening in individual and collective life.

Central to Rabinow and Rose's vision is the claim that today biopower is concerned principally with "our growing capacities to control, manage, engineer, reshape, and modulate the very vital capacities of human beings as living creatures" (Rose 2007: 3). This claim rests on two important observations. First, there has been a general shift in ways of governing in Western societies. According to Rose (2007), the ideal of the welfare state, dominant for much of the twentieth century, has generally yielded to that of the advanced liberal (or neoliberal) state. This new ideal is such that the political apparatus no longer appears obligated to safeguard the well-being of the population through maintaining a sphere of collective security. Social insurance—as an ensemble of state mechanisms that sought to insure individuals against the insecurities of social life—has thus largely given way to the privatized and individualized government of risk. Pragmatically, this has entailed, on the one hand, the parceling out (generally to the market) of many duties related to the administration of human health and welfare that previously had been the responsibility of the official state apparatus. Entities that Rose (2007) points to as now having important sway in the management of life include private corporations (transnational pharmaceutical companies and the biotech industry, for example), quasi-autonomous regulatory agencies (bioethics commissions), and professional organizations. On the other hand, the devolution of the state's powers has meant that individuals are now asked to take upon themselves the primary responsibility for managing their own security and that of their families. They are expected to adopt an entrepreneurial disposition toward life and insure themselves (using market mechanisms) against ill health, accidental loss, unemployment, and anything else that could potentially threaten their contentment. This emphasis on individual responsibility, Rose suggests, is particularly evident in the field of health, "where patients are increasingly urged to become active and responsible consumers of medical services and products ranging from pharmaceuticals to reproductive technologies and genetic tests" (2007: 4).

The second observation central to Rabinow and Rose's vision of biopower is that, as a result of developments in the life sciences, there has been a fundamental change in society's capacity to engineer human vitality (Rose 2001, 2007, Rabinow and Rose 2003, 2006). This change is essentially one of scale, involving moving from a molar to a molecular understanding of life. *Molar* refers to the body at the level of hormones, blood, tissues, organs, limbs, and so on. It is on the molar scale that the clinical medicine of the nineteenth and twentieth centuries sought to know and act on the body. The molar body, according to Rose, was the one "revealed to the gaze of the physician after death in the post mortem dissection, visualized in the anatomical atlas, accessed in life through any number of devices, starting with the stethoscope, that would augment the clinical gaze and allow it to peer into the organs and systems of the living body" (2007: 11–12). Although the molar level is still important in biomedicine today, Rabinow and Rose suggest that it has been supplemented, if not superseded, by a molecular vision of biological existence. As Rose puts it,

> life is now understood, and acted upon, at the molecular level, in terms of the functional properties of coding sequences of nucleotide bases and their variations, the molecular mechanisms that regulate expression and transcription, the link between the functional properties of proteins and their molecular topography, the formation of particular intracellular elements—ion channels, enzyme activities, transporter genes, membrane potentials—with their particular mechanical and biological properties. [2007: 12]

At the molecular level, life appears as a collection of intelligible vital elements that can be identified, isolated, controlled, mobilized, and reassembled. As such, life is no longer seen as natural or immutable destiny. Rather, as Rabinow and Rose (2003: xxxi) note, it is envisioned as artificial: as inherently manipulable and re-formable, open to calculative intervention and administration.

It is the complex of marketization, responsibilization, and molecularization that gives contemporary vital politics in the West its particular character. According to Rabinow and Rose (2003, 2006, Rose 2007), biopower today, with its emphasis on making life, is clearly visible in a number of basic ways. First, the object of contemporary biomedicine is no longer simply to cure illnesses and restore health. Rather, it is also to control and manage human biological processes in order to prevent disease, enhance health, and optimize the quality of one's existence. Second, individuals nowadays are increasingly relating to themselves in somatic terms, that is, as biological creatures. Many have thus come to define their citizenship not as a set of rights and duties tied to a nation-state but as an obligation to pursue life, health, and healing actively. Third, there has been a rise in new forms of somatic expertise—of multiple vocations that claim authority over and seek to manage particular aspects of biological life. These experts range from geneticists and specialists in reproductive medicine to stem cell therapists and bioethicists. Finally, over the past few decades, new circuits of bioeconomics have come into being. We are thus now witnessing, as Rabinow and Rose put it, "a large scale *capitalization of bioscience* and *mobilization* of its elements into new exchange relations: the new molecular knowledges of life and health are being mapped out, developed and exploited by a range of commercial enterprises, sometimes in alliance with States, sometimes autonomous from them, establishing constitutive links between life, truth and value" (2006: 203). From this perspective, then, biopower today is essentially about the administration and maximization of life. It is about how individuals—together with the doctors, scientists, entrepreneurs, and others who target life as a prime object of their knowledge and intervention—have made fostering biological existence a central stake in politics.

A Racial Politics of Life

Where can we locate the vital politics of racialized pharmaceuticals?[3] As I noted earlier, the present-day concern with the racialization of pharmaceuticals is partially tied to the ways in which race has historically been biologized. Beginning in the eighteenth century, as part of the more general effort to find order in

3 On biopolitics, race, and pharmaceuticals, see also Roberts 2011b, Krupar and Ehlers forthcoming.

nature, scientists have sought to use physical features—such as skin color, the shape of the face and skull, and hair form—to construct classificatory schemes of humankind (Stepan 1982, Omi and Winant 1994, Jackson and Weidman 2006). On the basis of skull formation, for example, the German physician Johann Blumenbach (1969) divided the human species into five varieties or races: Caucasian, Mongolian, American, Ethiopian, and Malay. Although such classificatory schemes were initially taken as referring to somewhat fluid biological groupings, by the nineteenth century they were seen as describing fundamentally distinct types of humans. Furthermore, individual racial groups came to be viewed as possessing different natural capacities: to reason, make moral judgments, attain civilized behavior, and so forth. Ultimately, they were ranked in relation to one another, with some groups deemed innately superior and others inferior. Specifically, racial scientists insisted on the essential superiority of white Europeans, distinguishing them from the "other" groups and effectively establishing a hierarchy in which physical markers came to designate the place a group occupied in social relationships. The scientific systems of classification advanced during the nineteenth century thus created seemingly immutable hierarchies based on the molar, phenomenal differences among humankind—that is, on the belief that certain physical traits are tied to attributes of behavior, intellect, and morality. As such, race was basically constructed as an essence, a natural, biological phenomenon whose meaning is prior to and beyond the reach of human intervention. Indeed, for racial scientists, race was destiny.

This biologically determinist way of thinking about race, which lasted in different guises well into the twentieth century, underpinned diverse but invariably exclusionary racial politics of life. The most notorious example is no doubt the eugenics project of Nazi Germany. The basic goal of the Nazi state, like that of other eugenic enterprises, was to create a new and better social order through fostering the vital qualities of the species body (Proctor 1995, Bauman 1989). Indeed, the supreme duty of Nazi political, medical, and other authorities was to secure the life of the people. Significantly, this eugenics project was very much a racialized one. Its focus was on the preservation of racial health. This entailed, on the one hand, cultivating the lives of those individuals deemed to be of healthy German racial stock and, on the other hand, the containment or elimination of any defective elements. It was thought that the propagation of the fit could really take place only through the systematic selection and elimination of any unhealthy threats (Bauman 1989). Among those targeted for exclusion and elimination were Jews. This population was typically characterized as a constitutively diseased race, as a cancer in the body of the German *Volk*. German scientists effectively constructed a worldview of Jews as racially predisposed to committing crime and to suffering from a host of other diseases, from mental illness to diabetes (Proctor 1995). Ultimately, such knowledge was used to justify the brutal mistreatment of Jewish populations: their segregation into crowded ghettos, imprisonment in concentration camps, and mass extermination. What the Nazi state did, then, according to Zygmunt Bauman, was "split human life into worthy and unworthy: the first to be lovingly cultivated and given *Lebensraum*, the other to be 'distanced,' or—if the distancing proved unfeasible—exterminated" (1989: 67–8). At work in Nazi racial politics was thus a blending of the management of life with the administration of death (Agamben 1998). It was in the name of preserving and fostering life that Nazi Germany was able to massacre millions of Jews.

In the United States, racial science has likewise buttressed exclusionary types of vital politics. During the 1920s, for example, the United States enacted a restrictionist immigration law (the Immigration Act of 1924) that severely curbed the flow of southern and eastern Europeans into the country. Driving the policy was the belief that immigrant groups such as Italians, Greeks, and Jews derived from inferior racial stock and were hereditarily predisposed to a host of deficiencies ranging from crime, pauperism, and feeblemindedness to epilepsy, tuberculosis, and insanity (Jackson and Weidman 2006).[4] Immigrants of such inferior stock, it was said, could only bring about the biological deterioration of the US population and weaken the nation's vitality. As noted eugenicist Lothrop Stoddard put it, "migrations of lower human types like those which have worked such havoc in the United States must be rigorously curtailed. Such migrations upset standards, sterilize better stock, increase low types, and compromise national futures more than war, revolutions, or native deterioration" (Stoddard 1921: 308). Another case in point is the history of medical experimentation on African Americans, most notably the Tuskegee Syphilis Study (Brandt 1978, Lombardo and Dorr 2006, Washington 2006). From 1932 to 1972, the US Public Health Service (PHS) experimented with some 400 poor African American males with untreated latent syphilis in order to determine the natural course of the disease. One of PHS's objectives was to test long-held scientific theories suggesting that venereal disease presents differently in blacks than in whites. As Harriet Washington notes, "PHS expected to validate its belief in a specific racial dimorphism of syphilis: Whereas the disease was thought to do its worst damage to the neurological systems and brains of whites, it was thought to wreak its worst havoc on the cardiovascular systems of blacks, sparing their relatively primitive and 'underdeveloped' brains" (2006: 156). When the study began, there was scant knowledge of successful treatments

4 The racial science of the early twentieth century constructed Europeans on the whole as superior to other racial groups (Africans, for example), yet among Europeans themselves there were hierarchies. Generally speaking, northern Europeans thought they were of better racial stock than southern and eastern Europeans (Jackson and Weidman 2006).

for syphilis. By the 1950s, however, penicillin had become widely accepted as an effective cure. Nevertheless, the study's subjects were left untreated and were actively prevented from seeking treatment outside the study, with tragic consequences. In the end, no fewer than 28 men, and possibly more than 100, died as a result of advanced syphilitic lesions. The Tuskegee men were thus effectively reduced to bare life: stripped of juridical protections, degraded to mere biological beings, and rendered disposable.

Given this history of exclusionary racial vital politics, it is understandable that there would be grave concern regarding the contemporary biologization of race. It is clear, however, that the life politics of racialized pharmaceuticals does not amount to a return to scientific racism. Indeed, we cannot simply locate this politics within the deterministic biology of the past. Rather, as Rabinow and Rose (2006) suggest, we must place it within the more complex biology of the present: a molecular genomic biology. Central to understanding the biologization of race today is the mapping of the human genome. In 2000, the Human Genome Project (HGP)—an effort coordinated by the US Department of Energy, the National Institutes of Health (NIH), and Celera Genomics (a private biotech company)—succeeded in sequencing the three billion base pairs that make up human DNA. The primary impetus behind this mapping was to search for ways to prevent, diagnose, and cure disease, that is, to improve human health (Duster 2006). The idea was that the decoding of the genome would permit scientists to identify human genes and thereby enhance our knowledge of the key biochemical processes of the human body and the genetic causes of disease.

In regard to the subject of race, the initial pronouncements following the sequencing of the human genome focused on the sameness of humanity (Lee 2006, Whitmarsh and Jones 2010). The sequence showed that humans share 99.9 percent of their genetic makeup, so HGP scientists proclaimed that human beings are essentially alike genetically and that racial differences have no bases in biology. However, other genomic researchers soon began to argue that even a 0.1 percent variation in genetic composition could translate into biomedically significant difference and that this variation noticeably maps onto traditional notions of race (Fujimura, Duster, and Rajagopalan 2008, Whitmarsh and Jones 2010). The current trend in genomic research is thus increasingly to focus on that small amount of genetic variation that separates one human being from another, with racial and ethnic categories, which are presumed to signify biological difference, serving as necessary variables (Lee 2006). Notably, the justification for this type of genomic research is still to enhance human health and vitality: knowledge of human genomic variation, particularly of racial and ethnic differences in disease susceptibility and drug response, is thought to be potentially valuable in making medical diagnoses and dispensing treatment (Fujimura, Duster, and Rajagopalan 2008).

This molecular reinscription of race (Duster 2006, Fullwiley 2007)—that is, the understanding of race at the level of genes and molecules—is in many ways fundamentally different from older molar visions of human difference. Today's scientific ways of thinking and intervening upon race do not by and large have domination and subordination as their end; they do not aim to set up immutable hierarchies of difference, discover essential racial truths, stigmatize individuals and populations, or legitimate inequality. Rather, their general principle is hope: hope that discovering the genetic factors underlying human disease might lead to interventions that will increase the health and well-being of racialized populations. The politics of race and genomics is thus grounded not in the negative, murderous underside of biopower but in its life-affirming pole. Indeed, as Rose argues, the politics of racialized medicine lies

> firmly within the transformed biopolitics of the twenty-first century. This is a biopolitics organized around the principle of fostering individual life, not of eliminating those that threaten the quality of populations; it is a biopolitics that does not operate under the sign of the sovereign state; it is a biopolitics that does not seek to legitimate inequality but to intervene upon its consequences. Crucially, it is a biopolitics in which references to the biological do not signal fatalism but are part of the economy of hope that characterizes contemporary biomedicine. [2007: 167]

What might be called the *molecular vital politics of race*, then, is about maximizing the quality of individual and collective life in all its difference. In today's configuration of knowledge and power, racial life is seen not as destiny, as a specific biological fate to which individuals are consigned, but as potentially malleable and open to various kinds of positive interventions and transformations.

To argue that the life politics of race today is not explicitly aligned with the death-making aspect of biopower is not to suggest, however, that it is free from ethical and sociopolitical problems. We can highlight three potential harms here. First, although it may be the case that contemporary racialized medicine does not seek to stigmatize individuals and populations, this does not mean it cannot. When a racially defined group is identified as having a higher genetic susceptibility to a particular disease, there is always a possibility that the group will be stigmatized. Early efforts to screen for sickle cell anemia, to highlight one case, resulted in the racialization of this disease as black, even though other subgroups also demonstrate high incidences of the condition. The outcome was that African Americans experienced substantial discrimination in employment and insurance (Wailoo 2001). That such a scenario could play out again is not out of the question. Second, even though racialized medicine might have as one of its goals the reduction of health disparities, it could also very well help reproduce inequality. For example, to the extent that too much weight is given to genetics as an explanatory factor in disease causality, the effect could be to minimize other, proven explanations of health disparities, namely the social and physical environment (Lee, Mountain, and Koenig 2001). To jettison the social as an explanatory mechanism would be to risk reproducing the very disparities one is trying to overcome. Third, although racialized medicine might be grounded in the life-affirming pole of biopower, fostering life is not necessarily always its primary concern. Research on race and genetics is increasingly taking place in a market context and thus is often subject to the demands of capital (Koenig, Lee, and Richardson 2008). This emergence of race as a potentially valuable genetic biocommodity means that in some cases making profits actually outweighs saving lives. Overall, then, although racialized medicine today is clearly on the side of life, it does have its own particular modes of exclusion.

A Map of the Book

This book is intended as a contribution to the rethinking of race and biopower in the genomic age. The argument I advance is that we need to locate racialized pharmaceuticals within the transformed biopolitics of the twenty-first century—a politics that clearly has life, not death, as its *telos*. Focusing specifically on BiDil, I suggest, on the one hand, that drugs targeted at particular racialized groups are ostensibly about fostering the vitality of the racial body. Indeed, on some level BiDil plainly aims to save lives and improve the quality of people's biological existence. As such, it is integrally connected to issues of rights and citizenship (Inda 2011). Racialized drugs are about the right of socially excluded populations to have access to the benefits of modern medicine. They are about the recognition of biological survival as a supreme value and the obligation to safeguard a person's bodily being. On the other hand, I also note that although drugs such as BiDil might help save African American lives and bring a measure of hope to a community that has historically been denied access to the benefits of modern medicine, we need to be mindful of the exclusionary vital politics of racialized drugs. Specifically, we must be careful not to obscure the social significance of race and reduce health disparities to health differences grounded simply in biology and genetics (Kahn 2005). We must also be wary of the stigmatizing potential of conflating race with biology. There is a danger with race-based medicine that, in neglecting the social and in biologizing race, medical and societal inequities will simply intensify. The point, then, is that although biopower in a genomic age might be focused on nurturing life and not be explicitly racist (in the sense of producing a division between those who must live and those who must die), it nevertheless has an underside. So, taking seriously the Janus-faced nature of biopower, I am concerned in this book with both the life-affirming aspects of racialized medicine and its potentially exclusionary vital politics.

Methodologically, the book relies principally on printed source materials—including government publications, scientific journals, archival documents, proceedings of scholarly conferences, newspapers, business reports, popular magazines, and published interviews with key stakeholders. The approach I take to these materials is ethnographic. My understanding of *ethnographic* is filtered through the work of Paul Rabinow. Discussing "society," he notes the following: "An ethnographic approach to society as the product of historical practices combining truth and power consists of identifying society as a cultural object, specifying those authorized to make truth claims about it and those practices and symbols which localized, regulated, and represented that new reality spatially (form is equally a cultural object)" (1989: 11). Similarly, I identify BiDil as a cultural object and use printed materials to pay close attention to the languages and voices of those authorized to make truth claims about racialized pharmaceuticals, as well as to explore the concrete practices that have given rise and shape to such drugs.

The trajectory of the book is as follows:

Chapter 2 provides a context for understanding the emergence of BiDil as a racial drug, focusing on two sets of factors. The first set consists of twentieth- and twenty-first-century developments in the biosciences, specifically the emergence of the field of pharmacogenetics and the mapping of the human genome. As a result of these developments, scientists, medical researchers, and politicians have come to believe firmly that notable differences exist between racial groups at the genomic level and that these differences are medically significant. In particular, they have come to accept as fact the idea that genetic differences between racially marked populations have a bearing on drug response. The second set of factors consists of governmental efforts to eliminate racial disparities in health. Over the last couple of decades, there has developed a strong political desire in the United States to lessen the burden of disease on minority populations, resulting in the implementation of key policy changes that have encouraged the use of race in medical research. In 1993, for example, the NIH Revitalization Act required the incorporation of women and minorities as subjects in medical research funded by the NIH. And in 1997, the FDA Modernization Act mandated the development of guidelines to include these populations in clinical trials. This chapter, then, focuses on the epistemological and political factors that facilitated BiDil's birth as a racial medication.

Chapter 3 suggests that the contemporary appeal of race in medicine needs to be understood in terms of citizenship. Across the world, rights and citizenship have come to be linked to matters of health, disease, and illness. Indeed, many citizenship projects have come to tie ideas about citizenship to beliefs about the corporeal, biological life of human beings. In the United States, biologically based citizenship projects have become an important part of the political landscape, with individuals and communities increasingly defining what it means to be a citizen in terms of their vital rights—their rights to life, health, and healing. I suggest that advocacy for BiDil, especially on the part of African Americans, is precisely about vital rights. It is about entitlement to health services, improving care, and hope for better treatment. It is grounded in the belief that the African American community, which has historically been excluded from the benefits of biomedicine, deserves access to life-saving medications. Central here is the idea that African Americans have particular health needs that might be genetically based, and that medications targeted at this population are essential to realizing the hope of finding cures and achieving healthy bodies.

Chapter 4 explores the problem of race and biology. Critics of BiDil have argued that the existence of such a drug, which is targeted only at African Americans, de facto legitimates the idea that races are biologically distinct entities—that blacks have particular, intrinsic biological attributes that function to differentiate them from other groups. Moreover, they claim that focusing too much on genetics as a root of health disparities and emphasizing race-targeted pharmacology as a solution to such inequities unnecessarily takes attention away from the social causes of diseases. Although the concerns raised in regard to BiDil are certainly serious, I suggest that neither the maker of the drug nor the medical scientists involved in promoting it advocate any kind of crude genetic reductionism. For example, in regard to health disparities, it is certainly the case that NitroMed has suggested a genetic basis for heart failure among blacks, but the company has not ignored social and environmental causes. At the same time, it is also clear that BiDil is not problem free. Scientifically, a wealth of evidence suggests that though there may be differences in how populations react to drugs, overall they tend to overlap significantly in their response. There is thus no reason to target drugs to specific populations.

Chapter 5 looks at the relation between racial life and capitalization. There is little doubt that the project of fostering life and health in the United States is intertwined with the production of wealth. Indeed, commercial considerations (the necessity of generating profits, for example) visibly shape the kinds of questions that biomedicine and the biosciences ask, as well as the types of problems on which they focus. Important players in the capitalization of life have been pharmaceutical companies. The drugs they produce are of course involved in the cultivation of life. However, the promise of profits is also clearly a factor propelling the manufacture of pharmaceuticals. In such a milieu, the racial body has emerged as a potentially important source of economic value. In the case of BiDil, there is no doubt that commercial factors were a driving force behind the racialization of the drug. The scientists who developed BiDil sought first to have the drug approved for the general population. When this effort failed, they went back to the data from their clinical trials, reanalyzed it along racial lines, and concluded that BiDil appeared to work better in blacks than in whites. So race came to matter only following the FDA's rejection. BiDil's rebirth as a racial medication, then, was as much about saving the drug and its potential profits as about saving black lives.

Finally, Chapter 6 locates BiDil and racialized medicine in the context of neoliberalism. In neoliberal societies, it has become standard to downscale the state with respect to the social protection of the population and to saddle individuals with the responsibility of safeguarding their lives against the insecurities of living. The result of this social abandonment has been to make life more precarious for marginalized populations. In this final chapter, I suggest that the promotion of BiDil and racialized medicine as a means to remedy the issue of health disparities may lead to the further neglect of poor and disfranchised minorities. Because genetic models of disease causality prioritize biological over social determinants of health, they have great allure in a neoliberal context. If maladies can be remedied through genetic technologies, then why worry about the social conditions that affect individual and collective health? Genetic medicine can thus serve as an excuse for the state to withdraw from providing social protection to its population, and to reduce health to a matter of personal responsibility that can rightly be attained only through procuring medical products in the marketplace. Racial medicine can be problematic, then, because focusing on genetics as a way of dealing with health disparities can lead to the disregard of social remedies. Such neglect of the social would likely result in the reproduction of health inequalities and not in their elimination.

Chapter 2
The Making of BiDil

BiDil is a fixed-dose combination of two generic drugs, hydralazine hydrochloride[1] and isosorbide dinitrate. Both generics are vasodilators that relax the smooth muscle in blood vessels and cause them to dilate. The result is that blood is able to flow more easily through veins and arteries, and thus the heart does not have to work as hard at pumping (NitroMed 2007a). As I have noted, BiDil was developed as a therapy for heart failure, a progressive, chronic disease in which the heart's muscle gradually weakens and little by little loses its capacity to pump enough blood to meet the body's metabolic needs (HSFA n.d.). This illness affects close to five million Americans, with an estimated 400,000 to 700,000 new cases diagnosed each year (HSFA n.d.). There is about an equal percentage of men and women, the majority being more than 65 years old, and roughly 750,000 are African American (Rosamond et al. 2007, NitroMed n.d.a).

Notably, although BiDil is indicated only for self-identified blacks, the drug did not start out as a racially specific medication. Dr. Jay Cohn, the University of Minnesota cardiology professor who created BiDil, and his colleagues tracked efficacy data by race from the very first trials that evaluated the components of the drug, the Veterans Affairs Vasodilator-Heart Failure Trials, or V-HeFT I and II (Kahn 2004). They did not, however, originally deem race to be a significant variable in BiDil's efficacy. This was quite evident during the drug's initial audience with the FDA. A few years prior to approving BiDil as a racial drug, the FDA had actually rejected it as a medication for the general population. In the course of committee hearings, only passing reference was made to race. Speaking before the FDA's Cardiovascular and Renal Drug Advisory Committee in February 1997, Cohn stated,

> The majority of patients [in V-HeFT I and II] were Caucasian. That is, about 70 percent of them in both trials, but there was a fairly sizeable number of African-Americans in the trial. We won't go into that, but we have much data comparing the Caucasian and African-American responses. [US FDA 1997a: 20–21]

Cohn did not "go into that" because he was undoubtedly operating according to the dominant "one size fits all" model of drug development, which suggests that

1 While the full name of the product is hydralazine hydrochloride, it is often referred to simply as hydralazine.

therapies will work on all patients regardless of racial background. The inclusion of African American subjects in V-HeFT I and II was thus inconsequential. The goal was to have the drug approved for heart failure sufferers in general. It was only after the FDA denied BiDil's initial application that there was a turn to race as a significant variable.

In this chapter, I provide a history of BiDil, focusing on how the drug came to be racialized. I suggest that the making of BiDil as a medication for African Americans has to be understood in light of a number of important epistemological and political developments. The epistemological developments are twentieth- and twenty-first-century advances in the knowledges of life. Specifically, the advent of pharmacogenetics and the mapping of the human genome have given credence to the idea that genetic differences between racially defined populations matter when it comes to drug response and bodily well-being. The political developments are the movements, beginning in the 1980s, to eliminate racial disparities in health. In particular, there has been a political effort, embodied in a variety of federal initiatives, to include minorities in biomedical research as a way to address health inequalities. In effect, then, this chapter tells the story of BiDil against the backdrop of the epistemological and political conditions that made the drug possible as a racial pharmaceutical.

BiDil's Birth

The birth of BiDil as a medication for heart failure can be traced to the 1970s (Cohn 2005). In 1973, Jay Cohn hypothesized in the journal *Circulation* that vasoconstriction—a narrowing of the blood vessels that restricts or slows the flow of blood—was an important factor in heart failure (Cohn 1973). The reigning assumption at the time was that the disease resulted primarily from abnormalities in the heart's pumping function and had little to do with peripheral circulation, or how well the blood moved through the body's vessels. On the basis of this hypothesis, Cohn and his colleagues (Guiha et al. 1974) theorized that vasodilators might be a promising treatment for heart failure. The standard treatment at the time was a regimen of digoxin, a drug that strengthens the contractions of the heart muscle, and diuretics, which help to manage blood pressure. These drugs did little, however, to ameliorate the suffering of people with heart failure and improve their condition (Rotman 2005: 62). The idea behind using vasodilators was that by dilating the blood vessels and making it easier for blood to circulate, the heart would pump more efficiently, thus potentially allaying the symptoms and progression of the disease.

Vasodilators were put to the test in two studies sponsored by the US Veterans Administration and led by Cohn—the aforementioned V-HeFT I and II. Neither trial, it bears emphasizing, was constructed explicitly around race and ethnicity. Each study enrolled both white and black patients (all men),[2] but the goal was to test the efficacy of vasodilators on the general population, regardless of race. In V-HeFT I, which lasted from 1980 to 1985, 642 men with damaged cardiac function who were undergoing conventional therapy with digoxin and a diuretic were randomly assigned to three treatment groups. One group received a placebo, another received the alpha-adrenergic blocker prazosin (a vasodilator), and the third received the drugs hydralazine and isosorbide dinitrate (H/I), the components of BiDil (Cohn et al. 1986). Prazosin, like the placebo, failed to produce positive results. V-HeFT researchers found, however, that "the addition of hydralazine and isosorbide dinitrate to the therapeutic regimen of digoxin and diuretics in patients with chronic congestive heart failure can have a favorable effect on left ventricular function and mortality" (1986: 1547). The second V-HeFT trial took place between 1986 and 1991. It compared the effects of H/I with those of enalapril, an angiotensin-converting enzyme (ACE) inhibitor, in 804 men taking digoxin and diuretic therapy (Cohn et al. 1991). ACE inhibitors, which are vasodilators that work to lower blood pressure by preventing the constriction of blood vessels, were at the time a new class of drugs that, like H/I, had shown promise in reducing the mortality rates and improving the quality of life of heart failure patients. The results of V-HeFT II revealed that while both H/I and enalapril were effective in lowering death rates, the latter performed significantly better. They also showed that H/I improved ventricular ejection fraction (the heart's pumping function) and exercise tolerance more than the ACE inhibitor (Cohn et al. 1991). On the basis of these findings, V-HeFT investigators reached the general conclusion that vasodilator therapy should be included in the standard treatment for heart failure. Furthermore, they proposed that, because H/I and enalapril had different beneficial effects, the two regimens might fruitfully be used in combination.[3]

Significantly, in 1987, while still conducting V-HeFT II, Cohn applied for a patent on a method of using hydralazine and isosorbide dinitrate to reduce mortality associated with congestive heart failure. In the description

2 The inclusion of only men in the V-HeFT studies can largely be attributed to the general culture of medical research at the time. As Steven Epstein (2007: 4) has noted, until recently the standard practice in medicine was to summarily exclude women, children, the elderly, and racial and ethnic minorities from clinical research. The assumption was "that the absence of these groups didn't matter much, because the findings from studying the 'normative standard'—middle-aged white men—could simply be generalized to the entire population."

3 Following V-HeFT II, ACE inhibitors went on to become a first-line therapy for heart failure, whereas the H/I combination came to be recommended for patients who did not tolerate or respond to these drugs (Kahn 2004).

of the patent, alluding to the results of V-HeFT I, he noted "that while no statistically significant reduction in mortality could be established using prazosin hydrochloride in vasodilator therapy in chronic congestive heart failure, a combination of hydrazaline hydrochloride and isosorbide nitrate has been formed [*sic*] to substantially and significantly reduce the incidence of mortality in such patients" (Cohn 1987). The US Patent and Trademark Office granted Cohn the patent in 1989, giving him a monopoly to market the H/I combination as a heart failure medication through 2007 (Sankar and Kahn 2005: 456). Cohn then turned around and, in 1991, licensed the patent to Medco, an emerging North Carolina-based pharmaceutical company. The idea behind licensing the patent was to use Medco's expertise in human pharmaceutical development to turn hydralazine and isosorbide dinitrate, which hitherto had been dispensed separately, into a single pill for easier administration and greater patient compliance (Medco 1991). Medco entered the agreement with Cohn on the understanding that the FDA might accept the V-HeFT I and II results as the primary basis for the submission of a New Drug Application (NDA) for a combined H/I product (Medco 1991).

Within a few years, Medco had successfully combined H/I into a single tablet and named the drug BiDil (Medco 1992). Subsequently, in 1996, the company submitted an NDA for BiDil to the FDA (PR Newswire 1996). Shortly afterward, in February 1997, the FDA's Cardiovascular and Renal Drugs Advisory Committee met to consider Medco's application. At the meeting, Cohn, who had been working with Medco on developing BiDil, sought to convince the committee of BiDil's efficacy, maintaining

> that there is a strong basis for approval of BiDil for congestive heart failure. That is, that the combination of hydralazine and isosorbide dinitrate exhibits a survival benefit compared to placebo; that it exhibits a strong trend for improved exercise tolerance versus both placebo and ... Enalapril ...; [and] that it produces a sustained improvement in ejection fraction. [US FDA 1997a]

The committee was not swayed, however. On a vote of nine to three, it recommended against approving BiDil for use in congestive heart failure (US FDA 1997b: 3). This is not to say that the committee saw no clinical benefits to BiDil. Rather, the problem was that the V-HeFT studies were devised not as new drug trials but simply to assess the theory that vasodilators were effective treatments for heart failure. As a result, the studies did not generate the kind of statistical data necessary to meet the FDA's standards for new drug approval. Indeed, their numbers were deemed simply too muddled to be interpreted "with any degree of certainty" (US FDA 1997b: 2), or as Ralph D'Agostino, a statistician and committee consultant, put it, the V-HeFT studies were "nice," but "there's so much going on that nothing really comes out clearly" (Reuters Health Medical

News 1997). Ultimately, on the basis of the committee's recommendation, in July 1997 the FDA issued Medco a "Not Approvable" letter stating that additional clinical research would be necessary (NitroMed 2005a: 10).

The Turn to Race

Although the FDA's decision was a setback, it would not spell the end of BiDil. The drug would experience a rebirth as a racial medication. Following the FDA's rejection, Medco decided not to pursue the development of BiDil and handed its intellectual property rights back to Cohn (Kahn 2004: 16–17). At this juncture, because the FDA had requested additional information in order to reconsider BiDil's NDA, Cohn, together with cardiologist Peter Carson and other colleagues, went back to reexamine the V-HeFT I and II data. As Jonathan Kahn (2004: 16) has pointed out, Cohn could have reanalyzed the data along a number of dimensions, none of which involved race. For example, in an article evaluating H/I's effects on exercise tolerance in persons with heart failure, V-HeFT researchers listed more than 20 baseline characteristics of the studies' patients—including age, history of alcohol use, and history of hypertension—that might influence response to therapy (Ziesche et al. 1993). Any of these characteristics could have been used as a primary variable in reassessing H/I's efficacy. In another piece that describes the V-HeFT studies, Cohn (1993) highlights the possibility that multiple determinants can influence therapeutic response. He asks, "Do women respond the same as men? Do individuals with coronary disease respond differently than those with cardiomyopathy? Does ventricular geometry influence the response to therapy? Are there biochemical or hormonal markers that will affect the response to a specific intervention?" (1993: VI-2). Some of these questions could likewise have been used to organize the retrospective analysis of the V-HeFT data. Ultimately, Cohn and his colleagues did not reanalyze the data along the dimensions identified in these articles. Instead, they focused on race.

Two important contextual factors explain why the V-HeFT researchers turned to race. The first factor has to do with developments in the knowledges of life. Researchers have long observed that humans differ from one another in how they react to drugs and other foreign chemicals. For example, in the early twentieth century, British physician Sir Archibald Garrod suggested that genetically-based differences in biochemical processes could be the reason for adverse drug reactions (Meyer 2004). Subsequently, researchers discovered (in 1932) that individuals differed in their inability to taste phenylthiocarbamide, (in 1956) that patients who succumbed to apnea when injected with succinylcholine during anesthesia were deficient in the enzyme butyrylcholinesterase, and (in 1957) that people with a genetic deficiency in *N*-acetyltransferase developed peripheral neuritis following therapy with isoniazid (Kalow 2006). Also, some scientists suggested that drug response differed not just between individuals but also between racially defined populations. For example, in a clinical trial conducted with soldiers during World War II, American physicians observed that only a small number of whites but roughly 10 percent of blacks developed acute hemolytic crises when administered standard doses of antimalaria drugs such as primaquine (Meyer 2004). These types of observations eventually led to the formation of the field of pharmacogenetics in the 1950s. Pharmacogenetics is, essentially, the "study of genetically determined variation in drug response" (Jones and Perlis 2006: 92). At the heart of the field is thus the idea that individuals vary in how they react to drugs and that this variation is genetically controlled. Specifically, genetic variation is held to affect how people metabolize drugs, how drugs work within bodies, and the rates at which products are expelled from the body (Hedgecoe 2004: 10).[4]

As the field developed in the 1950s and into the 1980s, pharmacogeneticists made a number of important general discoveries (Jones and Perlis 2006). In the 1950s and 1960s, for example, researchers showed that a family of enzymes now known as the cytochrome P450 system was responsible for the metabolization of the majority of medications. In the 1960s and 1970s, it was established, on the basis of twin studies, that genetics determined the metabolism of numerous drugs, including ethanol, phenytoin, desipramine, and nortriptyline. Finally, in the 1970s and 1980s, scientists described the genes involved in metabolizing important medications such as anticancer agents and the antihypertensive drug debrisoquine. As these general discoveries were being made, researchers were also reporting important differences in how racial groups metabolized drugs. Significantly, such reports were particularly prevalent in the field of cardiovascular medicine (Urban 2010). In the early 1980s, several studies suggested that there were racial differences in how subjects responded to antihypertensive drugs, with blacks experiencing a better response to diuretics than whites, and blacks having a more favorable reaction to beta blockers than whites (Johnson 2008). Furthermore, on the basis of literature produced during the 1980s and 1990s, it became generally understood that blacks did not respond to ACE inhibitors quite as well as whites (Kaufman, Nguyen, and Cooper 2010). One study suggested that in order for black patients to obtain a therapeutic response similar to that of whites, they had to be administered between two and four times the dose of the ACE inhibitor trandolapril (Weir et al. 1995). Another study indicated that the risk of ACE inhibitor-induced

4 Genetic variation thus accounts for the fact that some people, known as slow metabolizers, experience adverse reactions if administered a standard dose of a drug, while others metabolize the same dose so quickly that they do not attain any kind of medical benefit (Hedgecoe 2004).

angioedema was considerably greater in blacks than in whites (Brown et al. 1996). Thus, by the time Cohn and his colleagues reanalyzed the V-HeFT data, the idea that racial groups differed in their response to drugs, particularly those related to cardiovascular health, was well established.

The second contextual factor that explains why the V-HeFT researchers turned to race is the then-burgeoning political concern to reduce racial and gendered health disparities (Lee, Mountain, and Koenig 2001, Kahn 2004). In the early 1990s, the US Department of Health and Human Services (DHHS) released a report entitled *Healthy People 2000: National Health Promotion and Disease Prevention Objectives* (US DHHS 1991). The document details the health status of the US population and sets out the nation's public health goals and objectives for the 1990s. Noted in the report is that although very few health statistics in the 1980s took race and ethnicity into account, those that did left little doubt about the reality of racial health disparities. For example, black babies were two times more likely to die before their first birthday than white babies; the rate of AIDS among Hispanics was almost three times higher than that of non-Hispanic whites; the incidence of liver cancer among Southeast Asians was more than 12 times greater than in the white population; and among American Indians, diabetes was so common that in many tribes more than 20 percent of the members suffered from the disease (US DHHS 1991: 32–9). Significantly, the report suggested that attending to the well-being of disadvantaged population groups was necessary in order to improve the future health status of the nation:

> Achieving a healthier America depends on significant improvement in the health of population groups that now are at highest risk of premature death, disease, and disability. ... In most cases and for virtually all health risks, they are members of certain racial and ethnic groups, people with low income, and people with disabilities. Special attention is needed to close the gap that exists between the majority of the population and the various minority populations. [US DHHS 1991: 46]

Among the primary goals articulated in *Healthy People 2000* was thus the need to reduce and eventually eliminate the disparities in health status that exist among different US population groups. Whether the problem is chronic illnesses, unintentional injuries, or infectious diseases, it is important, the report determined, to make available the services necessary to bring about improvements in the circumstances of disadvantaged minority communities.

As part of this general effort to address the problem of health disparities, there also developed a movement to remedy the underrepresentation of women and minorities in clinical research (Epstein 2007, 2010). Specifically, in the mid-1980s, an eclectic group of reformers—including women's health and minority health advocacy organizations, biomedical researchers, politicians, drug company scientists, and federal health officials—began to advocate for equity in biomedical inquiry. They argued that the practice of employing mainly white, middle-aged males as research subjects and letting them stand in for all humanity was simply not appropriate. Their objection was based on the idea that because social differences are medically relevant, it is improper to extrapolate the results obtained from the study of one group to other groups (Epstein 2010). Ultimately, this advocacy for inclusion resulted in the creation of a series of federal laws, policies, and guidelines designed to ensure the incorporation of underrepresented groups in health care research. In 1993, for example, President Clinton signed into law the National Institutes of Health (NIH) Revitalization Act. The act requires the NIH to, among other things, include women and minorities as subjects in all medical research sponsored by the agency, as well as to ensure that clinical trials are "designed and carried out in a manner sufficient to provide for a valid analysis of whether the variables being studied in the trial affect women or members of minority groups, as the case may be, differently than other subjects in the trial" (NIHRA 1993). A few years later, in 1997, the Food and Drug Administration Modernization Act required the Secretary of Health and Human Services, in consultation with the director of the NIH and representatives of the pharmaceutical industry, to "review and develop guidance, as appropriate, on the inclusion of women and minorities in clinical trials" (FDAMA 1997).[5] Mandates such as these created an environment in which attention to women and racial minorities in medical research and the interpretation of clinical data become not only thinkable but also necessary.

Importantly, the racial and ethnic categories that came to be used in the efforts to eliminate health disparities and include minorities in medical research were derived from the US Office of Management and Budget (OMB). In 1977, the OMB issued Statistical Policy Directive No. 15, "Race and Ethnic Standards for Federal Statistics and Administrative Reporting," which provided "standard classifications for record keeping, collection, and presentation of data on race and ethnicity in Federal program administrative reporting and statistical activities" (US Census Bureau 2005). The idea was to produce a government-wide set of racial and ethnic categories that would allow Congress, the courts, and other governmental entities to monitor compliance with a variety of civil rights initiatives and the extent of racial inequality in the United States (Bliss 2012). For example, standard data on race would allow monitoring of the Voting Rights Act, equal employment opportunity and affirmative action programs, and racial disparities in education, housing, health care, income, and so forth.

5 Pursuant to these mandates, the NIH and the FDA have each issued detailed guidelines for the inclusion of women and minorities in clinical research and trials. See NIH 1994 and US FDA 2005c.

Directive No. 15 initially recognized four racial categories ("American Indian or Alaskan Native," "Asian or Pacific Islander," "Black," and "White") and two ethnic groups ("Hispanic origin" and "not of Hispanic origin"). Subsequently, in 1997, the categories were modified slightly: the "Asian or Pacific Islander" classification was split into two categories, "Asian" and "Native Hawaiian or Other Pacific Islander," and the "Hispanic" category was changed to "Hispanic or Latino" (OMB 1997). In promulgating its taxonomy, the OMB issued an important caveat: that the "classifications should not be interpreted as being scientific or anthropological in nature," but should be understood as sociopolitical constructs meant to advance social, cultural, and political goals (US Census Bureau 2005). When social categories are used in biomedical research, however, they are easily transformed into biological categories. The categories that came to be seen as vital to ascertaining and combating disparities in health were thus very much biologized social categories.[6]

It was in this epistemological and political context, then—with both research findings and political projects suggesting the need to take racial differences into account when considering matters of health—that Cohn and his colleagues went back to the V-HeFT data and reanalyzed it along racial lines. Their retrospective analysis, published as a paper entitled "Racial Differences in Response to Therapy for Heart Failure: Analysis of the Vasodilator-Heart Failure Trials," compared the responses to therapy of black (395) and white (1,024) patients in the V-HeFT studies (Carson et al. 1999). The researchers found that

> race impacts importantly on the mortality reduction observed with vasodilator and ACE inhibitor therapy. The H-I combination appears to be particularly effective in prolonging survival in black patients and is as effective as enalapril in this subgroup. In contrast, enalapril shows its more favorable effect on survival, particularly in the white population. [1999: 182]

Because the number of blacks in the V-HeFT studies was too small, Cohn and colleagues could not conclusively demonstrate that H/I worked better in blacks than in whites. They were, however, able to conclude that "the consistency of observations of a racial difference in response in V-HeFT I and V-HeFT II" lent "credence to the suggestion that therapy for heart failure might appropriately be racially tailored" (Carson et al. 1999: 186). In fact, they advised that whereas ACE inhibitors should probably remain the primary therapy for white patients, the H/I combination could prove to be an attractive alternative for black patients.

6 As I discuss in Chapter 4, although taking race into account is important for the elimination of health disparities, the use of social categories in biomedical research potentially geneticizes these categories, making disparities appear to be grounded in genetic difference rather than in social inequality (Roberts 2011a).

Ultimately, Cohn and his colleagues argued that their findings underscored the need to conduct prospective trials involving large enough numbers of blacks to clarify this population's response to heart failure therapies.

Encouraged by the findings of the retrospective analysis, Cohn continued his pursuit of bringing BiDil to market. His efforts focused on targeting the drug to African Americans. His thinking was that the FDA could be approached with the new information about BiDil's efficacy and be persuaded to consider the drug as a race-specific medication. One of Cohn's initial moves was to contact NitroMed, a Boston area biotechnology company specializing in nitric oxide-enhancing medicines, about taking on the development of BiDil (NitroMed 2005a: 16). After conducting its own reanalysis of the V-HeFT data, the company acquired the intellectual property rights to the drug in 1999 (PR Newswire 1999). In announcing the acquisition, NitroMed stated that it intended to amend the existing NDA for BiDil and seek an indication for the drug as a treatment for heart failure in African American patients. With this goal in mind, NitroMed and Cohn, who was serving as a consultant to the company, met with the FDA in 1999 and 2000 to explore further development of the drug (NitroMed 2005a). Following these discussions, in March 2001 NitroMed received a letter from the agency stating that "[g]iven the subset finding and the overall trend toward a survival effect in V-HeFT I, we believe a single, clearly positive study in a CHF [congestive heart failure] population would be a basis for approval of BiDil for the treatment of heart failure in blacks" (quoted in NitroMed 2005a: 11). In a second important move, Cohn and Carson filed a patent application on September 8, 2000 to use H/I in "treating and preventing mortality associated with heart failure in an African American patient" (Cohn and Carson 2000). The original general methods patent for BiDil was set to expire in 2007. So, by applying for a race-specific patent, Cohn essentially sought to extend BiDil's market protection. The reformulated patent, whose rights Cohn ultimately assigned to NitroMed, would give its holders exclusive rights to market the H/I combination to African Americans until 2020, thirteen years beyond the initial patent (Sankar and Kahn 2005: 458).[7] With the new BiDil patent filed and the FDA letter in hand, the stage was set for NitroMed and Cohn to launch the African American Heart Failure Trial (A-HeFT).

Begun in May 2001, A-HeFT was the first clinical trial focused strictly on African American men and women afflicted with heart failure (NitroMed 2005a, PR Newswire 2001). This historic study was cosponsored by the Association of Black Cardiologists (ABC), who helped NitroMed recruit patients and medical researchers (NitroMed n.d.b). A-HeFT was designed to determine the safety and efficacy of BiDil for self-identified blacks. One thousand and fifty patients with New York Heart Association heart failure classifications III and

7 The race-specific BiDil patent was ultimately issued on October 15, 2002.

IV (meaning moderate to severe) were randomized into two groups. One group received BiDil with a standard course of treatment, which generally included digoxin, diuretics, beta blockers, and ACE inhibitors. The other group was given a placebo in addition to the standard medication. A-HeFT was expected to last until 2005. However, its data and safety monitoring board, an independent group of experts assigned to monitor the trial, and its steering committee halted the study in July 2004 due to the "significant survival benefit" of BiDil (NitroMed 2007b). Results from A-HeFT indicated that, compared to the placebo group, individuals who took BiDil experienced a 43 percent decrease in the risk of mortality, a 33 percent reduction in the rate of first hospitalization resulting from heart failure, and a general improvement in their quality of life (Taylor et al. 2004). Shortly after the end of the trial, in December 2004, NitroMed completed the submission of a revised NDA for BiDil, seeking an indication of the drug for blacks only (NitroMed 2005a).

A Racial Drug

The Cardiovascular and Renal Drugs Advisory Committee of the FDA met to reconsider the application for BiDil on June 16, 2005. From the start, NitroMed was in a better position to have the drug approved than Medco had been eight years earlier. The main problem with Medco's NDA for BiDil, as noted earlier, was that the V-HeFT studies were not designed to meet the FDA's standards for clinical trials. As a result, the agency had deemed the V-HeFT statistics too messy to serve as the basis for endorsing the drug. By contrast, A-HeFT was designed explicitly to meet the FDA's criteria for new drug approval. Muddled statistics were thus not an issue. In fact, the FDA's statistician reports, which were completed about a month or so before the Advisory Committee met, generally supported the A-HeFT findings. For example, one report noted the following:

> The A-HeFT study was prematurely terminated for a significant reduction of mortality on BiDil. Even though less data than planned was collected as a result of early termination, A-HeFT was able to meet its primary endpoint of a significant favorable change in the mean of the composite score of mortality, first hospitalization for HF [heart failure] and QOL [quality of life] on BiDil compared to placebo. [Lemtouni 2005: 11]

A second report was likewise positive, stating that the "results of A-HeFT seem to provide support for the post hoc findings for black patients in V-HeFT I and II" (Hung 2005: 3). The general conclusion reached in the reports was thus that

BiDil could be safe and effective in African American individuals afflicted with heart failure.

Also strengthening NitroMed's position to have BiDil approved was the existing epistemological and political climate. In the years between Cohn's reanalysis of the V-HeFT data and the FDA's Advisory Committee meeting, the idea that genetic differences between racially defined populations mattered when it came to health received a significant boost due to the mapping of the human genome, and the elimination of racial health disparities became an even more central goal of political and medical authorities. As noted in Chapter 1, in 2000, the Human Genome Project succeeded in producing a rough draft of the human genome—that is, a preliminary map of the three billion base pairs that constitute human DNA. Eventually completed in 2003, the human genome map was touted as vital to discovering the genetic causes of disease and hence to the improvement of human health (Duster 2006). Importantly, although the initial declarations following the sequencing of the genome emphasized that all humans are essentially the same genetically, and thus that race has no basis in biology, some scientists soon argued that genetic variation between individuals, as small as it might be, was biomedically significant and generally correlated with traditional ideas of race (Whitmarsh and Jones 2010). A strong trend thus emerged in genomic research to focus on racial and ethnic differences in disease susceptibility and drug responses as a way to improve human health and vitality. For example, the International HapMap Project—a large-scale sequencing project started in 2002 to uncover the genetic causes of complex diseases such as heart disease, diabetes, and cancer—organized its collection and storage of data on the basis of population groupings that correspond to traditional racial taxonomies: Nigerian (African), European American (European), and Chinese and Japanese (Asian) (Hamilton 2008). In the field of pharmacogenetics, the NIH's Pharmacogenomics Research Network (PGRN), a nationwide collaboration of scientists who study how genetic variation affects drug responses, likewise stratified population samples by race and ethnicity in its research projects (Giacomini et al. 2007, Fullwiley 2007). An emblematic PGRN project is the Pharmacogenomics and Risk of Cardiovascular Disease (PARC) study. Using a cohort of 944 African American and European American subjects, the overall objective of PARC was "to identify genetic determinants of the wide range of interindividual variability in phenotypic and clinical response to statins" (Giacomini et al. 2007: 333).

While developments in genomics lent further legitimacy to the idea that genetic differences between racially defined populations are medically relevant, the continued focus on health disparities brought increased attention to the need to deal with the medical problems of racial minorities. In 2000, the DHHS released *Healthy People 2010*, a report updating the health status of Americans and the public health goals of the nation (US DHHS 2000a). The report notes that although strides had been made during the 1990s in improving the health of African Americans, Hispanics, American Indians, and Asians and Pacific Islanders, these racial minority populations still suffered disproportionately from a variety of maladies, ranging from heart disease, AIDS, and diabetes to cancer, tuberculosis, and hepatitis. As in *Healthy People 2000*, a principle goal articulated in the report was thus the elimination of health disparities. This goal was to be accomplished, in part, by working to expand minority access to quality health care. Notably, the effort to address the issue of health disparities continued to include a focus on remedying the inadequate representation of women and minorities in medical research. The efforts of the FDA were particularly significant. The same year that BiDil came up for approval, the agency released its *Guidance for Industry: Collection of Race and Ethnicity Data in Clinical Trials* (US FDA 2005c). The urge to collect data on race and ethnicity was based on the idea that racial groups potentially differ in how they respond to drugs. As the report notes,

> Differences in response to medical products have already been observed in racially and ethnically distinct subgroups of the US population. These differences may be attributable to intrinsic factors (e.g., genetics, metabolism, elimination), extrinsic factors (e.g., diet, environmental exposure, sociocultural issues), or interactions between these factors. For example, ... studies have shown that Blacks respond poorly to several classes of antihypertensive agents (beta blockers and angiotensin converting enzyme (ACE) inhibitors). ... Clinical trials have demonstrated lower responses to interferon-alpha used in the treatment of hepatitis C among Blacks when compared with other racial subgroups. [2005c: 3]

In stipulating the collection of racial and ethnic data, the FDA recommended that the pharmaceutical industry utilize OMB categories. Using standardized categories was seen as crucial to being able to evaluate any differences in the safety and efficacy of medicines among racial and ethnic groups.

Significantly, the political concern with health disparities and the epistemological emphasis on genomic differences ended up converging, creating a drive to promote genetic research as a way to alleviate inequalities in health. The activities of the NIH are instructive here. In 2002, the agency released its *Strategic Research Plan and Budget to Reduce and Ultimately Eliminate Health Disparities* (NIH 2002). The report noted that even after accounting for socio-environmental factors (socio-economic status and education level, access to and quality of health care, racial and ethnic discrimination, and cultural issues), racial disparities in disease susceptibility and responses to therapy persisted. Examining the role that genetics might play in explaining such disparities was thus deemed crucial. One of the key NIH entities that emphasized genetic research on health disparities was the National Human

Genome Research Institute (NHGRI). In its vision for the future of genomics research, the NHGRI identified as a grand challenge the need to develop "genome-based tools" that deal with health disparities and "improve the health of all" (Collins et al. 2003). To this end, the institute sponsored a number of initiatives focused on the genetics of health disparities, including the Africa America Diabetes Mellitus Study, the African American Hereditary Prostate Cancer Study Network, and the Study of Hereditary Hemochromatosis and Iron Overload Disease in Diverse Populations. Other NIH institutes likewise engaged, but to a lesser degree, in initiatives to determine the role of genetics in health disparities. For example, the National Institute of Diabetes and Digestive and Kidney Diseases was involved in a project to detect regions of the human genome that exhibited evidence for linkage in type 2 diabetes (NIH 2002), and the National Institute on Alcohol Abuse and Alcoholism named as a priority the identification of the biomedical, namely genetic, risk factors that contribute to disparities in the effects of alcohol (NIAAA 2002).

When BiDil went up for review, then, not only were the FDA's statistical reports favorable, but so was the political and epistemological climate, which encouraged solving the problem of racial health disparities through genetically inflected research. As I noted in Chapter 1, although all of the speakers at the public portion of the Advisory Committee meeting expressed support for the approval of BiDil, some suggested that it should be indicated for the general population and not just for blacks (US FDA 2005a). Their basic argument was that drugs worked on people regardless of race. Approving BiDil for a specific racial group was thus scientifically unjustifiable. Importantly, this argument was refuted by those who suggested that it was biologically plausible for there to be differences in how African Americans responded to BiDil and other drugs, and that this plausibility was enough to justify considering the medication for blacks only. For example, FDA Advisory Committee Chairman Stephen Nissen, speaking in reference to the Antihypertensive and Lipid-Lowering Treatment to Prevent Heart Attack Trial (ALLHAT), noted that "there was some pretty strong evidence in ALLHAT that there were [racial] differences in responses to this classification of drugs. So, yes, the road to hell is paved with biological plausibility but there is a biologically plausible explanation" (US FDA 2005a: 359). The case for approving BiDil for just blacks was bolstered by advocates in the African American community who saw the drug as a way for the FDA to remedy historical inequalities in biomedical research and care. For instance, Congresswoman Donna Christensen, a representative of the Congressional Black Caucus (CBC), stated,

> today, ladies and gentlemen, you have before you an unprecedented opportunity to significantly reduce one of the major health disparities in the African American community and, in doing so, to begin a process that will

> bring some degree of equity and justice to the American healthcare system. ... The position at the CBC on the approval of BiDil is clear and unequivocal. It should be approved and indicated for use in African Americans. [Christensen 2005: 202–3, 208]

In the end, the FDA Advisory Committee voted to recommend approval of BiDil, with seven members supporting the drug as a race-specific medication and two advocating that it be indicated for the general population (Nissen 2005).

Subsequent to the Advisory Committee's vote, the FDA officially approved BiDil for blacks only on June 23, 2005. In laying out the FDA's justification for approving BiDil as a race-specific drug, Robert Temple and Normal Stockbridge, both of whom were on the Advisory Committee, pointed to the evidence indicating the different impacts of BiDil on black and white heart failure subjects. As they put it, "there was very strong evidence that hydralazine hydrochloride–isosorbide dinitrate was extremely effective in self-identified black patients and considerable evidence that the effects were far smaller, if present at all, in white patients" (Temple and Stockbridge 2007: 57). Furthermore, Temple and Stockbridge signaled the significance of remedying the inadequate representation of black people and other populations in the drug development process, noting that "race and other demographic characteristics have long been important to consider in analysis of trials and as a matter of equity and justice" (2007: 59). They concluded by suggesting that "the FDA approval of a fixed combination of hydralazine hydrochloride–isosorbide dinitrate to treat heart failure in self-identified black patients was a scientifically reasonable, data-based decision, one that provided a major benefit in a group that is particularly burdened by congestive heart failure" (2007: 61). It was thus that BiDil became the first racial pharmaceutical. Its package insert reads, "BiDil is indicated for the treatment of heart failure as an adjunct to standard therapy in self-identified black patients to improve survival, to prolong the time to hospitalization for heart failure, and to improve patient-reported functional status" (NitroMed 2005b).

Conclusion

In this chapter, I have presented a history of BiDil, concentrating on the epistemological and political factors that facilitated the transformation of the drug into a racialized medication. In particular, I have noted how advances in the knowledges of life, namely pharmacogenetics and the mapping of the human genome, gave credence to the idea that race matters when it comes to disease susceptibility and drug response, while political concern with health disparities was drawing attention to the need to deal with the health issues of racial minorities. Such developments created a climate in which it was deemed legitimate to target a drug at African Americans in the name of equity and justice and on the basis of the belief that this group was somehow genetically different from other racial and ethnic groups. Importantly, this brief history hints at how BiDil is very much implicated in a racial politics of life. As I have noted, this is a politics that has as its aim fostering the biological vitality of the racial body. The story of BiDil specifically points to how problems of health and disease have become integrally connected to questions of rights and citizenship. Indeed, as a medication intended for a minority population, BiDil is, if anything, about vital rights. It is about entitlement to quality health care and medications as a way of nurturing the life of the black body. The next chapter takes up the subject of BiDil and citizenship.

Chapter 3
Biosocial Citizenship

Over the past few decades, as anthropologist Aihwa Ong (2006) has noted, health-based claims and matters of life have become central to the citizenship politics of the West. In France, for example, ill health is now by and large deemed the most credible grounds for conferring legal recognition upon asylum seekers, with individuals suffering from life-threatening pathologies the most likely to gain official residency permits (Fassin 2001, Ticktin 2011). In the Ukraine, the sickened bodies of Chernobyl nuclear disaster victims have served as the foundation for demanding access to biomedical resources and staking claims of citizenship (Petryna 2002). And in the United States, individuals afflicted with a wide range of diseases—from AIDS and mental illness to chronic fatigue syndrome and muscular dystrophy—are taking action and being recognized on the basis of their damaged biology (Rapp, Taussig, and Heath n.d., Landzelius 2006). Across the West, then, individuals have come to make claims on and be recognized by political, medical, and other authorities in terms of "their 'vital' rights as citizens" (Rose and Novas 2005: 441).

Significantly, pharmaceuticals play a central role in the politics of health and citizenship. Indeed, images of rights, duties, and social membership in the West are routinely associated with access to and consumption of pharmaceuticals (Petryna 2006, Pollock 2012). In Brazil, for example, the state has followed "a policy of biotechnology for the people" (Biehl 2007: 8), universalizing access to life-saving AIDS medication in the name of fostering the health of each and every individual. In the United States, the activism of patient groups was instrumental in the passage of the Orphan Drug Act of 1983, a law that uses a variety of economic and legal incentives to encourage the development of drugs to treat people suffering from rare and neglected diseases (such as Tourette syndrome, Wilson's disease, and myoclonus) (Novas 2009). Finally, in Barbados, where loss of workdays due to asthma puts a financial strain on the state, asthmatics have the right to free pharmaceuticals to treat their condition, with such entitlement carrying the political and moral responsibility to consume the medications judiciously in order to mitigate any economic burden to the nation (Whitmarsh 2009). So, not only are the vital rights of individuals being recognized, but pharmaceuticals have become key elements of that recognition.

In this chapter, I look at the connection between citizenship and pharmaceuticals, that is, explore the citizenship dimensions of BiDil. Specifically, I examine advocacy in favor of the drug, particularly by African Americans and NitroMed, in terms of what might be called *biosocial citizenship*. This is a form of citizenship in which individuals and groups are "made up"[1] and come together around a shared biological state or identification—a specific disease, corporeal vulnerability, genetic risk, embodied harm, somatic suffering, and so forth—in order to gain recognition, resources, and care. Biosocial citizenship thus amounts to collectivities mobilizing on the basis of their (damaged or precarious) biology as a way of securing vital rights—the right to life, health, and healing.[2] In the context of BiDil, African Americans have been "made up" and have come together around heart failure and the general suffering of the black body, the goal being to achieve access to the drug. African American biosocial citizenship is in this case about collective entitlement to health services, hope for better treatment, and helping suffering bodies. It is grounded in the belief that the African American community, historically excluded from the many benefits of biomedicine and thus disproportionately at risk of harm, deserves access to life-saving medications. Pivotal is thus the idea that medications targeted to African Americans are essential to materializing the hope of finding cures and achieving healthier bodies.

Biosociality and Citizenship

In his essay "Artificiality and Enlightenment: From Sociobiology to Biosociality," Paul Rabinow (2005) coins the term *biosociality* to capture how new genetic knowledges and technologies (for example, the mapping of the human genome, polymerase chain reaction, and so forth) are giving shape to novel practices of life. Specifically, biosociality is employed to name the way in which the new genetics is operationalizing nature in such a manner as to model it "on culture understood as practice" (2005: 186). The idea here is simply that, as a result of new understandings of vital processes at the molecular level, life (nature) has been opened to all kinds of calculated intervention and reformation. It is that human biological existence is no longer regarded as destiny or fixed endowment but as something artificial—an object to be known in such a manner that it is made amenable to being reworked. One important manifestation of biosociality that Rabinow discusses is the

1 Ian Hacking (1986) uses the term "making up people" to refer to how new kinds of persons are created or brought into being through scientific knowledge and practice. In this chapter, I am concerned with how people, specifically African Americans, are made up or constructed as biosocial citizens.

2 As I note later, although biosocial citizenship might be grounded in a shared biological state or identification, extrabiological factors, particularly medical neglect and exclusion, are also important to groups coming together as biocollectivities.

"formation of new group and individual identities and practices" (2005: 188) out of emergent genetic truths. He shows that, through advances in genetic screening practices, individuals can now be revealed to be at risk of developing certain genetic disorders. Significantly, these presymptomatic individuals, as well as those who are already suffering from particular genetic maladies, are joining together into groups to demand recognition and make claims on the use of biomedical research and technologies. For example, there are already "neurofibromatosis groups who meet to share their experiences, lobby for their disease, educate their children, redo their home environment, and so on" (2005: 188). It is not difficult to imagine, Rabinow suggests, other such genetics-based groups forming—groups that "will have medical specialists, laboratories, narratives, traditions, and a heavy panoply of pastoral keepers to help them experience, share, intervene, and 'understand' their fate" (2005: 188). Thus, as vital processes become an object of technical manipulation, we end up with the cultivation of new subjects who understand themselves through their biology and engage in all sorts of life practices aimed at fostering individual and collective health.

Notably, Nikolas Rose and Carlos Novas (2005) have taken up the notion of biosociality and interpreted it through the lens of biological citizenship. The latter term is used to "encompass all those citizenship projects that have linked their conceptions of citizens to beliefs about the biological existence of human beings, as individuals, as families and lineages, as communities, as population and races, and as a species" (2005: 440). According to Rose and Novas, biological citizenship has both an individualizing and a collectivizing dimension. It is individualizing in the sense that all sorts of authorities—from medical personnel and insurance companies to political powers and legal professionals—have come to understand individuals and have sought to shape their identities in biological terms, through categories such as the disabled, the chronically ill, the child with attention deficit hyperactivity disorder, the presymptomatic person, and so forth. Moreover, individuals themselves have come to self-fashion through active engagement with knowledge about their bodily materiality. Such individuals, as Rose and Novas note,

> use biologically colored languages to describe aspects of themselves or their identities, and to articulate their feelings of unhappiness, ailments, or predicaments. For example, they describe themselves as having high levels of blood cholesterol, as being vulnerable to stress, as being immuno-compromised, or as having an hereditary predisposition to breast cancer or schizophrenia. Such persons use those languages, and the types of calculation to which they are attached, to make judgments as to how they could or should act, the kinds of things they fear, and the kind of lives for which they can hope. [2005: 445–6]

This engagement with biological languages and the general concern with health and illness are part of a broader contemporary "regime of the self" in which individuals are admonished to maximize the quality of their lives through active self-promotion and acts of responsible choice (2005: 441). The ideal subject here is the rational, prudent, and entrepreneurial person actively making decisions about his or her conduct in the pursuit of self-improvement. Under such a regime, the expectation is that individuals will build the appraisal of health risks into their life planning—that is, they will think about the future and take sensible measures to protect themselves against ill health. What is more, individuals will learn to make claims on political, medical, and other authorities in terms of their vital rights.

As for the collectivizing dimension of biological citizenship, it involves the mobilization of groups and communities on the basis of shared somatic identifications. Rose and Novas refer to such communities—whether linked to race and ethnicity, hereditary lineage, family, collective biological suffering, or shared disease states—as "biosocial groupings" (2005: 242). It is this collectivizing dimension that is closely tied to the notion of biosociality. For Rose and Novas, biosociality is in fact the collective expression of biological citizenship. They basically understand the term as referring to forms of collectivization assembled around a common biological status, genetic or otherwise. Drawing on Rabinow, Rose and Novas suggest that "new forms of 'biosociality' and new ethical technologies are being assembled around the proliferating categories of corporeal vulnerability, somatic suffering, and genetic risk and susceptibility" (2005: 442). Put otherwise, the point is simply that biosocial groupings, as predicted by Rabinow, have become increasingly significant. From AIDS organizations and genetically-based groups to mental health associations, individuals are coming together on account of their biologies. Sometimes these biosocial groups are actual organizations whose members engage face to face at meetings or other events. Just as often, however, nowadays they are largely virtual communities linked through the Internet and e-mail. Whatever their mode of interaction, the citizenship practices of biosocial communities tend to be similar. Using AIDS collectivities as an example, Rose and Novas (2005: 448–9) note that such groups have a number of crucial citizenship functions: to disseminate information about their disease, to search for new types of treatment, to develop ways of managing the everyday effects of the disease, to lobby for rights and battle stigma, to aid those suffering from the illness, and to demand a voice in the creation and consumption of medical knowledge and expertise. This mobilization of biosocial communities in the name of health and illness is also part of the contemporary regime of the self. Such groups are essentially imagined as voluntary associations of active citizens—as biocollectivities brought together in self-interested pursuit of mutual benefits.[3]

Rose and Novas's engagement with the concept of biosociality is important in at least two respects. First, they significantly expand the purview of what counts as a biosocial group. Whereas Rabinow highlights the genetic basis of biosocial groupings, Rose and Novas (2005: 450) emphasize their sundry foundations, asserting that such collectivities are premised not just on genetics, but also on other biological conditions—conditions whose causes may be social, uncertain, or contested. The central feature of biosociality for Rose and Novas is thus not genetic commonality but the mere fact of shared biological injury. Indeed, it does not matter that the somatic affliction that brings a group together is not genetic in origin. What matters is simply that the group's members are united around common biological damage and suffering. The second important aspect of Rose and Novas's engagement with biosociality is the framing of the concept explicitly in citizenship terms.[4] The idea is that biosociality is not just about individuals forming groups on the basis of some sort of biological identification. It also entails, as we have seen, these biocollectivities mobilizing in order to gain access to vital rights and resources. Given this understanding of biosociality as categorically a form of citizenship, I suggest that an alternative and perhaps more appropriate name for the concept might be *biosocial citizenship*. This term captures how biosociality fundamentally involves the linking of collective rights to matters of health, disease, and bodily suffering. Indeed, it highlights the intimate coupling of biosociality and citizenship—how groups seek to legitimate rights in the name of their biologically damaged and suffering bodies.

Racial Biosocialities

How can the concept of biosociality or biosocial citizenship be used to think about African Americans and BiDil? Generally, I suggest that modes of group identification based on race and ethnicity are central to understanding the making of biosocial collectivities (see also Gibbon and Novas 2008). The idea is that although biosocial groupings do in fact form around specific genetic or disease conditions, from muscular dystrophy and Huntington's disease to bipolar disorder and PXE (pseudoxanthoma elasticum), they frequently do

3 See Rose 1996a for a more detailed discussion of the contemporary emphasis on governing through community.

4 Rabinow (2005) does discuss how afflicted individuals gather into groups to lobby for their diseases. However, he does not frame this advocacy or activism in citizenship terms.

so in contexts where racial (and other) identities are potent galvanizing forces (Tutton 2012). So, although biosocial groups might generally form irrespective of race, they are also often organized explicitly around racial and ethnic lines. Indeed, race and ethnicity are routinely implicated in the formation of biosocial groupings. We might call such biocollectivities based on race *racial biosocialities*.

An excellent example of racial biosociality is the Ashkenazi Jewish population in the United States. This community has long been associated with particular genetic maladies, now often referred to as *Jewish genetic diseases*, including Tay-Sachs disease (TSD), Fanconi anemia, Canavan disease, and familial dysautonomia. Through this strong association with genetic disease, Ashkenazi Jews have been mobilized as a community of shared biological identification (Rose 2007). In the 1970s, for instance, Jewish families, religious groups, and community organizations lobbied for and embraced—in the name of Jewish survival and self-preservation—mass genetic screening and reproductive counseling as techniques to prevent the birth of babies with TSD (Wailoo and Pemberton 2006). TSD is a lethal genetic disorder in which the nervous system is progressively destroyed, generally resulting in death by the age of five. It is passed down within families in an autosomal recessive fashion, meaning that one must inherit two copies of the defective gene, one from the mother and one from the father, in order to have the disease. Scientific developments during the 1970s produced no effective therapies for TSD but led to advances in prevention, which essentially entailed identifying carriers of TSD through genetic testing and presenting them with appropriate information regarding the possibility of their children having the disease. Given the absence of suitable treatments, the most effective strategy for the Jewish community to deal with TSD thus became prevention. Testing campaigns took place in religious institutions and colleges, single people and potential spouses were encouraged to find out if they were TSD gene carriers, and couples who each carried a copy of the gene were warned about the risk of giving birth to a TSD child. In effect, American Jews were able to mobilize as a biosocial community and use genetic knowledge about the risk of disease to develop programs that allowed them to make decisions regarding reproduction and potentially alleviate the pain and suffering that came with having a Tay-Sach's baby. Today, with so-called Jewish genetic diseases continuing to be a salient aspect of Ashkenazi life, American Jews persist in organizing on the basis of their damaged biology. A number of organizations, including the Victor Center for the Prevention of Jewish Genetic Diseases in Philadelphia and the Center for Jewish Genetics in Chicago, are at present devoted specifically to managing such diseases.

It is likewise the case that African Americans have been mobilized as a biosocial community. This mobilization is quite evident in regard to sickle cell anemia (SCA), a life-threatening, autosomal recessive genetic disorder wherein a person's red blood cells, which are normally flexible and round, assume a rigid, sickled (crescent) shape. These abnormal cells can hinder the ability of blood, and hence oxygen, to circulate throughout the body. The symptoms and complications of SCA include swollen hands and feet, frequent infections, delayed growth, vision problems, stroke, pulmonary hypertension, organ damage, and most characteristically, "sickle cell crises"—periodic episodes of acute and unpredictable pain affecting different parts of the body, typically the bones, joints, legs, arms, lungs, and abdomen. For most people, there is no cure for the disease. So, having SCA often means lifelong suffering and premature death. Although the disease affects a number of populations in the United States, it is most commonly associated with African Americans.[5] Indeed, historically, this population has been disproportionately encumbered with SCA. Significantly, in 1971, in an effort to mitigate the burden of sickle cell suffering in the black community, the Black Panther Party launched a campaign to combat the disease (Nelson 2012). A central premise of the campaign was that the prevalence of sickle cell anemia among African Americans was a function not simply of genetic inheritance but also of social factors, namely the intentional and pernicious neglect of this population and its maladies by the US medical establishment. The campaign was designed to counter this neglect. Specifically, it sought to challenge health inequality by furnishing African Americans with access to medical services: health education about SCA and its transmission, as well as free genetic screening to test for the disease and for carrier status. The hope was that by dealing with the societal harms that facilitated the persistence of sickle cell anemia and aggravated its effects, the Panthers would go a long way toward reducing incidences of the disease. Through its activism, then, the Black Panther Party constructed African Americans as a biosocial community entitled to health care rights in the name of their biologically injured and suffering bodies.

Importantly, the Jewish and African American examples just presented indicate that racial biosociality arises not simply out of a shared biological state, but also out of extrabiological factors.[6] Indeed, though these groups may form in relation to the biological body, it is clear that socio-environmental influences also play a decisive role in making them come together (see Wehling 2011). In the case of Jewish Americans, for example, their biosociality is tied not just to Jewish genetic diseases, but also to the shared experience of social, political, and

5 Sickle cell anemia is most common among populations who live in or trace their ancestors to the malaria belt regions of Africa, southern Europe, the Middle East, and South Asia. Scientists believe that the sickle cell mutation developed as an evolutionary response to malaria. People with only one copy of the gene mutation, though not immune to the disease, have an increased resistance to it.

6 It is undoubtedly the case that extrabiological factors are key to the formation of biosocial groups more generally. See Wehling 2011 and Tutton 2012.

economic persecution and to the desire for Jewish survival and self-preservation. As for African Americans, their biosociality is linked not simply to sickle cell anemia but as well to the common experience of social marginalization and biomedical neglect, and to the yearning for justice and inclusion. Central to racial biosociality are thus questions of injustice, inequality, and discrimination. These commonalities are just as important as biology to racial groups uniting as biosocial collectivities.

BiDil and African American Biosocial Citizenship

I suggest that the case of African Americans and BiDil represents another important example of racial biosociality and shows how both biological and extrabiological influences shape biosocial group formation. Through various types of knowledge, scientific and other experts have constructed African Americans as a community of shared biological identification that is suffering from a malady, heart failure, that requires a specific medical intervention, namely BiDil. Moreover, African Americans themselves have come to self-fashion in terms of their corporeality and have made claims on both political and nonpolitical authorities as a biocollectivity entitled to vital rights. Notably, the call for African American vital rights is grounded not just in the precarious biology of this population but also in the shared experience of biomedical neglect—the experience of being denied access to the advantages of biomedicine, and the way in which this exclusion contributes to the production of their biological problems. My concern here, then, is with the understanding of African Americans as a biocollectivity with rights to biomedical attention. It is with the promotion of BiDil as essentially a biosocial citizenship project—with how the drug is implicated in the making of claims, to the right of health and healing, on behalf of and by African Americans.

The analysis presented here has two strands. The first strand focuses on the making of African Americans as a biosocial community, highlighting the role that precarious biology, medical neglect, and the experience of bodily pain and suffering play in the coming together of this population as a biocollectivity. The second strand deals with the promotion of BiDil as a technology of hope—as a drug that will alleviate African American suffering. In discussing these two strands, I draw attention to the actors involved in constructing African Americans as a biosocial group and calling for their vital rights. These actors include NitroMed (as well as the scientists affiliated with the company) and a host of African American and other minority civil, political, and professional organizations, notably the Congressional Black Caucus, the National Association for the Advancement of Colored People (NAACP), the National Minority Health Foundation, the Association of Black Cardiologists

(ABC), the International Society on Hypertension in Blacks, and the National Medical Association.

Making a Biosocial Community

Central to the construction of African Americans as a biosocial community, I suggest, has been the fact of biological damage and the experience of biological suffering. Put otherwise, the biologically damaged and suffering body has been a crucial source of legitimacy for African American access to health care rights. Biology alone has not been enough, however, to bring African Americans together as a biosocial group. Also central has been the experience of biomedical neglect. Thus, both biological and extrabiological factors have been crucial to the fashioning of African American biosociality. Specifically, on the one hand, African Americans have been constructed as a community of shared biological identification that is disproportionately afflicted—compared to other populations—with heart failure. Importantly, the etiology of heart failure, whether genetic or otherwise, matters less than the sheer fact of biological damage. On the other hand, African Americans have been perceived as neglected by the medical establishment and thus as excluded from the benefits of modern medicine. This biomedical neglect is believed to take two forms: first, a lack of available effective medications for African Americans; and second, this population's limited access to health care.

The most important dimension of African American biosociality is no doubt the precarious or damaged biology of this population. Indeed, the wounded body has served as the principal tie bringing African Americans together as a biocollectivity. A key actor in the construction of blacks as a biologically injured and suffering population has been NitroMed, the maker of BiDil. From the outset, the company has been concerned with presenting its interest in the drug as connected to the need to relieve the collective and individual suffering of African Americans that results from biological damage. Many of its publications indeed stress how blacks are disproportionately afflicted with heart failure, and the burdensome nature of this disease. For example, in its 2003 annual report, NitroMed notes:

> Heart failure—or end-stage cardiovascular disease—affects approximately five million Americans. There is no cure for this disease and more than 50% of patients die within five years of diagnosis. African Americans suffer a disproportionate incidence of cardiovascular disease. With respect to heart failure, they are affected at a rate almost twice that of the corresponding white population and are more likely to die from it. [2004: 2]

A now discontinued website created by NitroMed called Heart.Health.Heritage went even further in pointing out just how severely heart failure affects African

Americans. On a page entitled "Risk to African Americans," the company stated the following:

> Although heart failure is on the rise all across America, it hits the African American community hardest. In the United States, African Americans are 50% more likely to develop heart failure than the general population. African Americans tend to develop heart failure at an earlier age than other Americans. The symptoms of heart failure tend to be more severe and to worsen more quickly in African Americans. More African Americans are hospitalized than other Americans. [NitroMed 2006a]

The portrait that NitroMed paints is thus of a community of suffering. It is a picture of African American sociality formed around biological distress.

NitroMed has not left the experience of biological damage and suffering at an abstract level, however. The company has notably sought to ground the pain of heart failure in very specific black bodies. The FDA testimony of Debra Lee (see Chapter 1), whose trip was financed by NitroMed (Lee 2005: 218), is indicative of this effort. But Debra's story is not the only one that NitroMed spotlights. In the company's 2004 annual report, we read the third-person accounts of two other patients who participated in A-HeFT. The first story is that of Dianna Wells, a 51-year-old woman from Dallas, Texas:

> At the young age of 47, Dianna saw the first signs of heart failure when she had difficulty breathing and experienced extreme fatigue and swelling. Confused by the symptoms because she was normally an active, fit person, her condition deteriorated so rapidly that she could no longer work. Dianna's clothes became tight due to the swelling, and she was forced to wear a larger shoe size. She could not even do the little things that most people take for granted, such as walking, vacuuming the house or even talking on the phone for long periods of time. Several months later—and one trip to the local emergency room—Dianna was diagnosed with heart failure. [NitroMed 2005c: 4]

The second story recounts the experience of Leland Ramey, a 56-year-old man from Cincinnati, Ohio:

> Leland can remember being on business trips and unable to make it through a day without experiencing extreme exhaustion. At first, he tried blaming his fatigue on flying or the sub-zero temperatures of Chicago, but became frustrated when he had to cut short many evenings with clients and co-workers. An avid runner, Leland spent much of his time training for marathons and was confused by his lack of energy and difficulty walking. In 1995, Leland was diagnosed with heart failure after suffering a mild stroke and discovering a potentially fatal blood clot

> in his leg. Over the next year and a half, Leland struggled just to make it through the day, and because of his heart failure symptoms was forced to discontinue his work as a chemical engineer for Proctor & Gamble. [NitroMed 2005c: 6]

What these two stories highlight is the individual experience of affliction—how biological damage and suffering are inscribed on particular African American bodies.

Besides NitroMed, a host of African American organizations—most notably the ABC and the NAACP—have been involved in the construction of blacks as a biologically injured population. The ABC is a professional organization devoted to reducing disparities related to cardiovascular disease in racial minority populations; the NAACP is a grassroots group dedicated to civil rights more generally. Both organizations have been very strong supporters of BiDil and, like NitroMed, have stressed the taxing effects of heart failure on the African American community. For example, Keith Ferdinand, a cardiologist and chief science officer of the ABC, stated the following:

> Heart failure is a major health concern in the US and is particularly problematic in the African-American community where the disease has an earlier onset and exhibits increased mortality, even with hospitalization. Early onset is manifested primarily in middle-aged patients, ... with a higher mortality than in whites. Between the ages of 45 and 64, African-American males have a 70% higher risk for heart failure than Caucasian males. African-American females between the ages of 45 and 54 have a 50% greater risk to develop heart failure than Caucasian females. It is estimated that there are approximately 700,000 African-Americans with heart failure and the number is expected to grow to 900,000 by 2010. [Ferdinand 2006a: 86]

The NAACP has made complementary claims. Juan Cofield, president of the New England Conference of the NAACP, has emphasized that "[c]ardiovascular disease disproportionately affects African Americans, and access to [BiDil] will help to alleviate the burden of this disease" (Business Wire 2007).

Notably, the ABC and the NAACP have been concerned not just with black suffering due to heart failure. For them, this disease is just one of many maladies that disproportionately affect African Americans. Speaking at a 2007 press conference entitled "The Healthcare Quality Crisis in America: A 21st Century Civil Rights Priority!" Hilary Shelton, director of the NCAAP's Washington Bureau, asserted, "African Americans are 23% more likely to die from various types of cancer than Whites. African American and American Indian/Alaskan Native infant mortality rates are more than 2 times higher than those for their Caucasian counterparts. ... African American diabetics are more than 3 times more likely than Caucasian diabetics to have a lower limb amputated"

(PR Newswire 2007). Heart failure is thus located as part of a broader pattern of African American biological damage and suffering.

In addition to highlighting the damaged biology of African Americans, NitroMed, the ABC, and the NAACP have also focused on the question of biomedical neglect. Indeed, African American biosociality is founded not simply on the damaged biology of this collectivity, but also on the common experience of biomedical abandonment. NitroMed's main concern has been the lack of effective drugs to treat African American heart failure. In a 2005 briefing document prepared for the FDA, the company notes:

> Current treatments for black patients with heart failure are insufficient. Published data suggest that ACE inhibitors may be less effective in black patients, and may cause higher rates of angioedema in this population. Beta blockers have generally not been tested in a meaningful number of black patients with heart failure; in addition, when used in the treatment of hypertension, beta blockers have a known attenuation of effectiveness in black patients. [NitroMed 2005a: 10][7]

This lack of suitable medications for treating African Americans who have heart failure is a claim that NitroMed and its scientists repeat over and again in company documents, scientific papers, mass media interviews, and conference presentations. For example, Michael Loberg, then president and CEO of NitroMed, speaking at the Deutsche Bank Securities 29th Annual Health Care Conference, asked, "[A]re the African-American patients somewhat underserved by existing heart failure medication?" His answer:

> Here's what the FDA has said over the last 20 years. The first package insert up here is Vasotec. It's from the early 1980s. ... And it says that in controlled trials of Vasotec and ACE (ph) inhibitors in general that the effect on blood pressure in African-Americans was reduced and that the incidences of angioedema, the life-threatening adverse reaction, are higher. ... If you look at a more recent package insert, this is from 2003, the next one Cozaar, Losartin [*sic*]. The life study looked at patients with hypertension and it asked the question could Losartin reduce the incidence of stroke? And what it said was that, yes, in the overall population,

7 One of the main sources of this claim is a 2001 paper published in the *New England Journal of Medicine* that compares the response of blacks and whites to ACE inhibitory therapy (Exner et al. 2001). The study found that although the ACE inhibitor enalapril proved valuable in reducing the risk of hospitalization for heart failure among white patients, the drug did not have a similar beneficial effect on African Americans. For a critique of the idea that ACE inhibitors work substantially better in whites than in blacks, see Sehgal 2004.

> it did. But in the African-American sub-population, it did not, that there were [*sic*] no evidence of benefits. In fact, the patients, the African-American patients on Losartin slightly worsened and that the FDA could find no other basis, other than race. [FD Wire 2004]

The implication here is that African Americans constitute an underserved population when it comes to medicines for heart failure, and that pharmaceutical companies and the medical establishment have generally failed to address the cardiovascular health needs of this population.

The ABC and the NAACP have similarly emphasized that medications for heart failure do not appear to work well on African Americans. For example, the NAACP, in a resolution encouraging black patients with heart failure to ask their doctors about BiDil, notes that "some medicines approved for the treatment of heart failure, such as ACE inhibitors, appear to be less effective in Black patients" (NAACP 2005a). And Malcolm Taylor, chair of the ABC Heart Failure Committee, states that "African-Americans may also be underserved in heart failure because some existing drugs, such as ACE-inhibitors and ARBs, approved for use in heart failure, may be less effective in African-American patients under certain conditions. These ethnic differences are documented in package inserts for enalapril (Vasotec), and for losartan (Cozaar), indicating less favorable outcomes in African American patients" (Taylor n.d.). For these African American organizations, however, the problem of black health does not stop at the unavailability of effective medications for heart failure. More so than NitroMed, they have been broadly concerned with the African American community's general lack of access to health care. The NAACP's Health Department, as a case in point, has highlighted that minorities are less likely to be insured than nonminorities, that they tend to receive substandard medical care, and that they often have limited access to mental health services (NAACP n.d.). And the ABC, in a report on cardiovascular health disparities coauthored with the National Institutes of Health, likewise highlights the inequalities in the health care system: "Structural factors and inequities in health care resources may hamper African Americans in gaining access to quality care. Large numbers of African Americans receive care in urban medical centers or community clinics. In both types of settings, resources may be lacking to deliver the high level of care required for good outcomes" (ABC and NIH 2004: 10). Black suffering is thus as much about lack of access to health care as it is about the unavailability of effective drugs.

The Biochemical Materialization of Hope

Significantly, the construction of African Americans as a wounded biological community has served as a basis for making biosocial citizenship claims.

Indeed, the belief that blacks suffer disproportionately from heart failure and that current therapies do not work well on them has underpinned calls for access to rights. The particular rights in question amount to the availability of biomedical cures. Specifically, they mainly involve access to BiDil. The drug has essentially been promoted as offering hope to a suffering population underserved by the medical-pharmaceutical establishment. This biochemical materialization of hope has at least two significant, intertwined dimensions. First, it is about saving African American lives and improving the quality of existence for individuals. The message is thus that the illnesses of African Americans are worthy of being treated, that black lives are worth saving. Second, the promise of BiDil is more generally about reducing health disparities, about eliminating the inequalities that exist between blacks and other populations in regard to cardiovascular health. The gist here, then, is that the wounded and suffering black body has served as a key source of legitimacy for gaining rights, with BiDil materializing the hope for longer and healthier African American lives. Without a doubt, access to pharmaceuticals has become entwined with the prospects of health and happiness.

A central actor in the biochemical materialization of hope has, not surprisingly, been NitroMed. The company has not only helped to create a picture of black suffering, but has also proposed a solution to the problem, namely BiDil. NitroMed has indeed been very keen to promote the drug as an antidote to the heart failure issues of the African American community. According to Michael Sabolinski, a former chief medical officer of NitroMed (2006–07), one of the main reasons the company focused its drug development efforts on African Americans was "healthcare disparities" (Johnmar 2006). He further notes that "[b]lacks tend to have more severe forms of heart failure and are twice as likely to die from the condition than whites. Despite this, there weren't any heart failure drugs being studied in an African American population." In this context, BiDil gets presented as a promising medication. As Manuel Worcel, another former NitroMed chief medical officer (1997–2006), puts it, "BiDil will provide new hope to black heart failure patients who suffer a disproportionate burden of this disease" (NitroMed 2005d). The foundations of this hope are the results of A-HeFT. Across numerous platforms, NitroMed has touted that the trial demonstrated BiDil to be a life-saving and life-enhancing drug. On its Heart.Health.Heritage website, for example, the company promoted BiDil as the "first treatment specifically for African Americans with heart failure," highlighting how this treatment has proved to be very effective:

> In a large clinical study, called the African American Heart Failure Trial (A-HeFT), a group of African Americans with heart failure took BiDil along with their usual heart failure medicines. Compared to a similar group of patients—taking only

> their usual medicine—39% fewer of the BiDil users required hospitalization for heart failure. And 43% fewer of the BiDil users died during the course of the study. The BiDil group also reported a significant improvement in their day-to-day functioning. [NitroMed 2006b]

BiDil is thus presented as a medication that helps a population very much in need of suitable therapy for heart failure. The drug promises to ease the collective suffering of African Americans, and to lead, perhaps, to a reduction in health disparities.

In addition to touting the alleviation of collective suffering, NitroMed has also promoted individual patient outcomes. This can be seen clearly in the patient profiles discussed earlier. Following her diagnosis of heart failure, Dianna Wells searched the Internet for information on heart failure and its treatment options. As a result of this research, she learned about A-HeFT and subsequently joined the trial in March 2003. The results of Dianna's participation in A-HeFT, according to the NitroMed narrative, were impressive:

> Since participating in the trial, Dianna has been able to start working again, part time. She can walk, go shopping, go up and down stairs and even vacuum. Her swelling has gone down substantially, and she has returned to her normal shoe size. For the first time in a long while, Dianna feels like she is able to live life fully again. [NitroMed 2005c: 4]

Leland Ramey's story presents a similar conclusion. He joined A-HeFT in late 2003 and experienced a significant improvement in his quality of life:

> Although he can no longer train for marathons, Leland is now able to walk more and keep in shape.
>
> During the trial, Leland experienced a decrease in his symptoms of fatigue. Now, with more energy, he can spend quality time with his kids, and he is able to return to many of the things he used to do before being diagnosed with heart failure. Leland is grateful for the opportunity to participate in the A-HeFT trial and the difference he believes it has made in his life. [NitroMed 2005c: 6]

BiDil thus not only gives hope to African Americans as a population, but also promises to relieve individual suffering and enhance the quality of black lives.

African Americans have likewise been key players in the biochemical materialization of hope. Indeed, a number of African American organizations have been involved in achieving the rights and fulfilling the hopes of African Americans through their advocacy efforts in support of BiDil. They have essentially drawn on the biology of African Americans in order to make citizenship claims. During the FDA Cardiovascular and Renal Drugs Advisory Committee meeting to discuss BiDil, for example, a number of African American organizations, including the Congressional Black Caucus, the National Minority Health Foundation, the ABC, the International Society on Hypertension in Blacks, and the National Medical Association, spoke in favor of the drug. Their remarks generally focused on the benefits of BiDil, particularly its life-saving qualities. Gary Puckrein, for instance, speaking on behalf of the National Minority Health Foundation, noted, "As evidenced by the A-HeFT results, approval of BiDil will have an immediate and positive impact on the health and quality of life of many patients with heart failure. ... I support BiDil because it will extend the life of many Americans with heart failure. I support it because it will improve the quality of life of these patients" (Puckrein 2005: 211–12). Dr. Charles Curry, from the International Society on Hypertension in Blacks, echoed this sentiment: "I don't think we really know for sure how the drug works, but what we do know is that there is a 43 percent reduction in mortality. Any doctor who treats sick patients cannot turn away from that" (Curry 2005: 233). This espousal of BiDil ultimately culminated in rather forceful calls for the FDA committee to approve the drug. As Lucille Perez, representing the National Medical Association, put it, "Given the disproportionate impact of cardiovascular disease on African Americans, anything short of approval cannot be justified. ... The National Medical Association urges this committee to recommend to the FDA that BiDil be approved. ... African Americans continue to die ... from heart disease at the alarming rate of 78,000 a year. This number could be significantly reduced if BiDil is brought to market as soon as possible" (Perez 2005: 258–9). For these African American organizations, then, BiDil offers the black community the opportunity to achieve a measure of health. They place substantial faith in the promise that biochemical technologies will prolong the lives of African Americans and help alleviate health inequalities. The drug thus essentially functions to materialize hope. It is seen as a means to achieve vital rights for African Americans and to relieve their biological suffering.

It should be noted, however, that although BiDil was important to the hopes of these African American organizations, the drug was only a part of their broader advocacy efforts focused on social justice in health care.[8] These organizations, along with others (notably the NAACP), took part in the aforementioned press conference, "The Healthcare Quality Crisis in America: A 21st Century Civil Rights Priority!" (PR Newswire 2007). Held on September 27, 2007, this conference generally drew attention to the lack of equality in

8 I should note here that NitroMed has also been involved in broader efforts to reduce health disparities. In 2005, for example, it partnered with the NAACP to develop health advocacy initiatives designed to promote equal access to quality health care (NAACP 2005b). However, more so than African American organizations, NitroMed has centered its health disparities efforts on BiDil.

health care and challenged the American medical system—doctors, insurance companies, and so forth—to take responsibility for the poorer health status of minorities. Moreover, the participants, calling health care the next civil rights battleground, vowed to work in concert on a series of projects designed to help build an infrastructure of health care research, financing, and delivery with the ability to provide high-quality care to all Americans. Among their first initiatives was Community HeartBEAT, an education and advocacy effort to reduce the morbidity and mortality rates of African Americans who have heart failure by improving physician quality of care and increasing patient knowledge about treatment options (PR Newswire 2007). Beyond their collective work, each participating organization has developed its own health advocacy projects. The ABC, for instance, has a program called CHOICES that trains lay health promotion specialists to screen clients for cardiovascular health problems such as obesity, hypertension, diabetes, dyslipidemia, and so forth. In 2005, more than 3,800 individuals were screened through this program and more than 14,000 received information about cardiovascular conditions (Williams 2007: 310). The NAACP has created such projects as Kick the Habit, a smoking cessation program focused on educating minorities about the perils of smoking (NAACP 2006). The general health goals of this civil rights organization are to "ensure access to high-quality affordable healthcare," "eliminate disparities in HIV/AIDS," "reduce disparities in respiratory diseases," promote "the development of good mental health practices and programs," and "reduce obesity disparities and related disease—diabetes, hypertension, heart disease" (NAACP n.d.). Although BiDil may be important, it is certainly not the only mediator of hope.[9]

Conclusion

The central claim of this chapter has been that BiDil is deeply implicated in a politics of health and citizenship. Indeed, the biosocial citizenship politics of the drug have been a central dimension of its social life. It is a politics in which recognition from and demands on political and other authorities are based on the vital needs and suffering of the black body. It is a politics wherein African Americans' biological status has been mobilized in order to gain access to rights. For a community historically neglected by pharmaceutical companies and biomedical authorities, the recognition of their biological suffering is an important achievement. Through BiDil, African American heart failure patients have been given hope that their suffering can be relieved. They have

9 Advocacy for BiDil can also be understood as part of a long history of African American health activism. See Nelson 2012.

been offered the prospect that their lives can be prolonged. Of course BiDil does not address the social and economic problems that many see as the root of black biological suffering (see Roberts 2011b). Indeed, as Didier Fassin (2001: 7) notes, contemporary recognitions of the suffering body tend to have the effect of reducing human existence to its mere physical expression and of imposing "a legitimate order defining citizenship on purely physiopathological grounds." But BiDil was never intended as a solution for all African Americans' problems. The drug's biosocial citizenship politics are actually more modest. African American supporters of BiDil are well aware that the drug is only a biological fix. BiDil's promise is thus simply to help prolong life and relieve biological suffering.

Chapter 4
Enlightened Geneticization of Race

Although the citizenship dimensions of BiDil have been significant, the drug has not been without controversy. In fact, it has been involved in a bitter debate over the meaning of race in genetics. Critics of BiDil argue that the existence of such a drug, one targeted at a particular population, de facto legitimates the idea that races are genetically distinguishable entities—that African Americans have intrinsic biological attributes that function to differentiate them from other groups (Kahn 2004, Roberts 2011a). They also claim that focusing too much on genetics as a root of health disparities and emphasizing race-targeted pharmacology as a solution to such inequities takes attention away unnecessarily from the social causes of diseases. At issue for these critics is thus the likelihood that striving for health equity by treating the racial body as a genetic entity will lead to the naturalization of health disparities, permitting biological explanations to overshadow social, economic, and ecological understandings of disease. Moreover, they fear that medical and societal inequities will simply intensify with the advent of race-based medicine.

In this chapter, I focus on such claims about the geneticization of race through BiDil—on how the scientific and institutional practices surrounding the drug have worked to inscribe race as a genetic fact. There is no doubt that the concerns raised regarding BiDil are serious. I suggest, however, that the proponents of the drug—whether NitroMed and its scientists, the FDA, or African Americans themselves—do not generally advocate any kind of crude genetic reductionism. The genetic inscription of race can in this case be seen as akin to what Adam Hedgecoe (2001) calls "enlightened geneticization." Writing in reference to mental illness, he notes that the discourse of schizophrenia genetics generally presents "current genetic thinking as reasonable, non-extremist, and accepting a rôle for non-genetic factors in schizophrenia causation" (2001: 875). Simultaneously, though, Hedgecoe argues subtly, this discourse "ensures that schizophrenia can only be considered in terms of *some* necessary genetic aetiology (even if it is not sufficient)" and "suggests that the variety of different possible environmental factors should be seen against a 'genetic baseline' which is the only single necessary condition for causation" (2001: 885). "Enlightened geneticization" is thus a nondeterministic type of geneticization that presents a complex, multifactorial vision of disease causation that does not reduce diseases or disorders to genes but makes a place for social and environmental influences. Ultimately, however, enlightened geneticization privileges genetic explanations and subtly diverts attention away from the nongenetic factors that contribute to ill health.

The geneticization of race through BiDil can likewise, if not exactly in the same way, be thought of as enlightened. It is enlightened simply in the sense that BiDil advocates generally present a complex, nonreductionist view of race and genetics. I suggest that although African Americans have no doubt been geneticized through the drug, this geneticization does not necessarily imply that races are discrete biological entities or that health disparities are simply genetic in origin. Indeed, most proponents of BiDil seem to be very well aware that race is a rather imprecise marker for genetic differences among populations and that inequalities in health cannot be reduced to genetics. At the same time, there are problems with how African Americans are geneticized through the drug. Supporters of BiDil may generally have complex views about the relation between race and genetics, but the fact that the FDA approved BiDil for just African Americans does give the impression that blacks constitute a distinct genetic population. In addition, although advocates do take into account the role of social factors in disease causation, they still generally support genetics as a way of addressing health disparities; a line of research that is not likely to be productive given that environmental determinants such as unsafe living conditions and inadequate access to health care clearly explain most health inequalities. What might be called *enlightened racial geneticization* thus provides a nonreductionist but nevertheless problematic understanding of race and genetics.

Race and Geneticization

To begin unpacking the geneticization of race through BiDil, let me place the drug in the context of the broader tendency in contemporary scientific practice to geneticize race.

There is no doubt that there is a strong propensity in today's scientific culture to think of race as a genetic fact. Central to this geneticization has been research in population genetics. Some population geneticists have argued that the mapping of the human genome has affirmed that the human population can generally be divided into five genetic groups that correspond to the major geographic regions of the world. In one influential study, for example, Noah Rosenberg and his colleagues (2002) examine the DNA of 1,056 individuals sampled from 52 populations around the world as a way of ascertaining the genetic structure of the human population. On the basis of their data, they make two important arguments. First, they suggest that all human populations are genetically similar, with intrapopulation genetic variation—that is, variation within any given population grouping—accounting for most human genetic diversity. Specifically, they note that "within-population differences among individuals account for 93 to 95% of genetic variation," whereas "differences among major groups constitute only 3 to 5%" (Rosenberg et al. 2002: 2381). Second, Rosenberg and his colleagues argue that although all humans are essentially alike genetically, it is possible to cluster them into subgroups based on allele frequencies—the degree to which variant forms of particular genes appear in a population.[1] The basic proposition here is that "genetic differences among human populations derive mainly from gradations in allele frequencies rather than from distinctive 'diagnostic' genotypes" (Rosenberg et al. 2002: 2384). In the end, using the software program *structure*, which utilizes genotype data to investigate population structure, the researchers identify six main genetic clusters, five of which coincide with the geographic regions of Africa, Eurasia, East Asia, Oceania, and America.[2] The significance of this study is thus that it gives credence to the idea that race is a genetically meaningful category. Indeed, by mapping genetic difference onto classical racial divisions based on continental ancestry, the study essentially constructs race as a genetic fact.

Building on the findings of population geneticists, some medical researchers have argued not only that race is biologically real, but also that the genetic differences that exist between racial groups are medically significant (Fausto-Sterling 2004, Braun 2006, Rose 2006). Such researchers have consequently highlighted the necessity of conducting genomic research on the relations between race, disease susceptibility, and drug response. Prominent among those who have emphasized this need are noted medical geneticist Neil Risch and his colleagues. In a number of papers, they have argued that race is an indispensable variable in genomic research (Risch 2000, Risch et al. 2002, Burchard et al. 2003). Their argument essentially has three main elements (Braun 2006). First, they make a case for the pervasiveness of population-specific risks of disease, highlighting how alleles pertaining to disease susceptibility and treatability occur at different rates in different populations. Second, they contend that research in population genetics has "proven" human beings to be biologically divided into five races, "defined on the basis of the primary continent of origin" (Risch et al. 2002: 3): African, Caucasian, Pacific Islander, East Asian, and Native American. Third, they argue that because these continental races generally

1 An allele is "the alternative form of a gene or DNA sequence that occurs at a given locus. Some loci have only one allele, some have two, and some have many alternative forms. Alleles occur in pairs, one on each chromosome" (Goodman, Moses, and Jones 2012: 246).

2 The sixth cluster generally consists of individuals of the isolated Kalash group, an Indo-European language population from northwest Pakistan.

match up with US Census racial categories, and hence with how individuals in the United States self-identify, then self-reported race is a good predictor of genetic constitution and must be incorporated into medical genetics research. Risch and his colleagues' basic argument, then, is that "information about patients' ethnic or racial group is imperative for the identification, tracking, and investigation of the reasons for racial and ethnic differences in the prevalence and severity of disease and in responses to treatment" (Burchard et al. 2003: 1174). To ignore race in genetic studies, they suggest, would be detrimental to the health of racial minority populations.

The challenge of taking race into account when conducting genetic research has been taken up by numerous scientists, resulting in a proliferation of what Steven Epstein (2007) calls "difference findings," some of which involve racial differences in disease susceptibility. Indeed, medical researchers have linked racial disparities in incidences of disease—from AIDS, breast cancer, and diabetes to prostate cancer, addiction, and lung cancer—to genetic variation (Lee, Mountain, and Koenig 2001, Frank 2001, Happe 2006, Epstein 2007, Wailoo 2011). An example is racial differences in breast cancer. Statistics show that African American women bear a disproportionate burden of the disease (Happe 2006). Although their lifetime risk of developing breast cancer is actually lower than that of white women, they are more likely to die of the disease (Krieger 2002). In 1998, for example, the breast cancer mortality rate for African American women was 28 percent higher than it was for white women (Jones and Chilton 2002: 540). African American women also tend to be diagnosed with breast cancer at a younger age, and often with more aggressive tumors and at a later stage of the disease (Trock 1996, Happe 2006). While some researchers have suggested that racial differences in disease manifestation and outcome are likely due to socio-environmental determinants (lack of access to medical care and environmental racism, for example), others have maintained that social causes cannot adequately explain such differences and therefore that genetic susceptibility must be a factor (Happe 2006). Researchers making the case for genetics have suggested, for example, that BRCA1 gene mutations "may contribute to breast cancer in a significant proportion of African-American women" (Olopade et al. 2003: 237).[3] Moreover, they have proposed that common variations of the genes that influence the metabolism of estrogen and environmental pollutants may function as disease risk factors in this population (Ishibe et al. 1998, Guillemette et al. 2000). These claims that genetics can account for breast cancer in African American women essentially suppose that race is a biological risk factor for disease.

3 BRCA1 is a well-known tumor suppressor gene. In normal cells, it helps prevent uncontrolled cell growth. Mutations of this gene, as well as of BRCA2, have been linked to hereditary breast cancer.

Difference findings also involve racial differences in response to medical treatment. In the field of cardiovascular health, as I noted in Chapter 2, there have been repeated claims that diuretics, ACE inhibitors, and other antihypertensive drugs work differently in black populations than in non-Hispanic white populations. These assertions about racial differences in drug response have not stopped at cardiovascular medications, however. According to geneticists Sarah Tate and David Goldstein (2004), claims have been made in peer-reviewed scientific journals about differences among racial groups in either the safety or efficacy of at least 29 drugs. Many (about half) of the drugs on their list are for cardiovascular conditions, but also included are medications for diabetes, hepatitis C, mental illness, pain relief, and so forth. The belief that pharmaceuticals work differently depending on the population that takes them thus holds true across an array of drug classes. Notably, the studies that Tate and Goldstein discuss tend to attribute racial disparities in drug response to differences in biological processes, including those involving genes. We can use medications for hepatitis C and pain as examples. First, a study comparing antiviral therapy for hepatitis in African Americans and non-Hispanic whites found that the former had a lower or poorer rate of response to treatment (De Maria et al. 2002). The study concluded that both environmental and genetic factors might be involved in the impaired ability of African Americans to overcome hepatitis C virus infections. Second, a research study that focused on evaluating ethnic differences in response to morphine determined that American Indians are more susceptible than Caucasians to morphine ventilatory depression—a decrease in the normal respiratory rate that can be harmful (Cepeda et al. 2001). It suggested that genetic variations in the enzymes that metabolize drugs account for racial differences in response to morphine. These contentions about differences in responses to drugs essentially presume that medically meaningful genetic variations exist among racialized groups.

BiDil and Genetic Fact Making

Today, then, there is a strong penchant in scientific thought for geneticizing race. Indeed, population geneticists and medical researchers have essentially constructed race as a genetic fact. The case of BiDil very much contributes to this scientific understanding of race. Through this drug, NitroMed, African American scientists, and the FDA have all been involved in the practice of geneticizing African Americans. These actors have made claims concerning racial differences in both disease susceptibility and response to medical treatment. Specifically, they have suggested that African Americans are genetically more susceptible to developing heart failure and that BiDil's efficacy in this population is likely connected to their biology.

Key to the geneticization of African Americans through BiDil has no doubt been NitroMed. The company has repeatedly claimed that the reason African Americans suffer disproportionately from heart failure, perform poorly on ACE inhibitors, and do well on BiDil might originate, at least partially, in genetics (NitroMed 2005a: 14–15). Such assertions turn on nitric oxide (NO), a chemical compound that forms in the endothelium (the cells lining the inner walls of blood vessels). NO, the production of which is believed to be largely genetically determined, has been found to be a central player in the dilation of the blood vessels. NitroMed has suggested that African Americans may be more likely than other groups to have an impaired ability to produce NO and thus to maintain open blood vessels. Ultimately, this dearth in NO production is deemed to predispose African Americans to develop heart failure. As NitroMed has put it, "The high prevalence of deficient nitric oxide-mediated vasodilation in black patients may explain in part why heart failure develops disproportionately in black patients" (NitroMed 2005a: 15). That BiDil, as opposed to other heart failure medications (such as ACE inhibitors), works well on African Americans has also been associated with nitric oxide. BiDil is believed to be an NO enhancer (NitroMed 2007a). One of the drug's components, isosorbide dinitrate, releases nitric oxide at the blood vessel wall. However, NO degrades rather quickly after its formation. Hydralazine, BiDil's other element, is said to prevent this degradation, thus leading to the enhanced presence of NO in the body. This increased availability of nitric oxide that results from the use of BiDil is deemed responsible for relieving the symptoms of heart failure in blacks.

Significantly, NitroMed has worked to link the efficacy of BiDil in African Americans explicitly to genetics. As part of A-HeFT, NitroMed conducted a substudy called Genetic Risk Assessment in Heart Failure (GRAHF) (NitroMed 2007c, McNamara et al. 2009). It compared the incidence of genotypes related to cardiovascular disease in 358 A-HeFT patients to the frequency of the same genotypes in white heart failure subjects who took part in the University of Pittsburgh's Genetic Risk Assessment of Cardiac Events (GRACE) trial. The goal was to determine whether genetic variations related to cellular levels of NO production influence an individual's response to BiDil. Central to the study was the endothelial nitric oxide synthase (NOS3) gene, which encodes the NOS3 synthesizing enzyme, the source of most endogenous vascular NO. Certain variants of the NOS3 gene are thought to reduce NO production in endothelial cell culture and thus lead to increased risk of coronary disease, hypertension, and stroke (McNamara et al. 2009). NOS3 is also believed to affect the therapeutic effectiveness of antihypertensive drugs. NitroMed presented its preliminary results as follows:

> Endothelial nitric oxide synthase (NOS3) gene researchers found that a majority of black patients in A-HeFT possess a specific gene variation that was observed in less than half of the white cohort from GRACE. NOS3, which encodes the nitric oxide synthesizing enzyme in the heart and vasculature, is important in hypertension and heart failure. The benefit of BiDil therapy on ... mortality, first heart failure hospitalization and patient functional status ... was seen in those possessing the specific NOS3 gene variation. [NitroMed 2007c]

The suggestion here is thus that BiDil's power to improve the condition of heart failure sufferers is related to a genetic trait that might be more common in blacks than in whites.

Following NitroMed's lead, African Americans themselves have likewise been implicated in the process of geneticization. Particularly important in this process has been the Association of Black Cardiologists (ABC). A number of medical researchers and clinicians affiliated with the organization have been involved in pointing to the role of genetics in heart failure and drug efficacy. Notable among these are Clyde Yancy, currently chief of the division of cardiology at Northwestern University's Feinberg School of Medicine, and Keith Ferdinand, Chief Science Officer of the ABC. Through the ABC, both were involved in A-HeFT and have served as advocates for BiDil. Of the two researchers, Yancy has probably been more associated with the geneticization of African Americans. He has repeatedly argued that "heart failure in Blacks is likely to be a different disease" (Black Issues in Higher Education 2002: 26) and that this difference is probably "physiologic" in nature (Yancy 2002: 218). By physiologic, Yancy essentially means genetic. As he puts it:

> The physiology of the heart and blood vessels may differ, and there may be certain other differences that are determined by variation in genetic signals. Much work needs to be done in this area, but there is growing curiosity that a genetic basis may exist to explain some of the differences in outcomes that are seen in Black patients with heart failure. [Black Issues in Higher Education 2002: 26]

Keith Ferdinand has made similar genetic claims. He has suggested that genetic variation might explain why standard heart failure therapies are less effective for blacks. In doing so, like NitroMed, he underscores the nitric oxide deficiency theory of black heart failure. Ferdinand notes:

> Based on the pathophysiology of HF [heart failure], blacks demonstrate less ability for endogenous nitric oxide to dilate peripheral blood vessels. This may be related to an increased frequency of genes that decrease the synthesis of nitric oxide in black persons. ... Black patients, therefore, may have a

decreased response to neurohormonal drugs such as ACE inhibitors, ARBs, and b blockers and an enhanced response to drugs that increase the delivery of nitric oxide. [2006b: 157]

Although both Yancy and Ferdinand speak in tentative language, using words such as *likely* and *may*, it is nevertheless clear that, for them, genetics plays a role in black heart failure and response to pharmaceuticals.

Finally, the FDA has also played a strong role in the geneticization of African Americans. Generally speaking, the approval of BiDil for just blacks certainly gives the impression that there is something biologically different about this population. Otherwise, why was the drug not approved for everyone? More specifically, the FDA, through its spokespeople, has indicated that it believes racial differences in drug response are connected to genetic differences. For example, Dr. Steven Nissen, who chaired the FDA's Cardiovascular and Renal Drugs Advisory Committee that recommended approval of BiDil, unequivocally made a case at the committee's hearings for using self-identified race as a surrogate for genetic differences. He stated:

You know, what do we try to do when we sit here at this committee? We try to identify whether a drug is efficacy [*sic*] and the population which the drug will benefit. We look at evidence. When the overwhelming evidence that leads me to believe that this drug [BiDil] is effective comes from a population that we can define by some characteristic—now, it is self-identified race in this case. That is very unusual. It is precedent setting. But it is the case. And we are moving forward in medicine toward the era of genomic-based medicine. There is no question that in 10 or 15 years it is going to happen. We are going to have the ability to look for a snip that tells us that this group of people will benefit from X drug or will be harmed by Y drug. I know it has been predicted for a long time and hasn't happened yet but it is going to happen, trust me.

So, what we are doing here is we are using the background, that being from the African Continent and immigrating to the United States, although often not voluntarily; that the population that comes from that ethnic background seems to have some differences. We already know that there are differences. We already know that. We know, for example, that ACE inhibitors don't seem to work as well in African Americans. We know that certain diseases are more prevalent or less prevalent. So, what we are doing is we are using self-identified race as a surrogate for genomic-based medicine and I don't think that is unreasonable. I wish we had the gene chip. I wish we could do it on a genetic basis. But, in the absence of that, we have some information that suggests that African Americans—we know that African Americans, self-identified, get a pretty robust response to the drug. [Nissen 2005: 354–6]

Nissen has suggested here that the ideal approach would have been to find the genetic markers related to BiDil's efficacy and then to target the drug to individuals with those specific markers, irrespective of race. However, given that the genomic sciences were not yet able to pinpoint these markers, it was reasonable to employ self-identified race as an imperfect stand-in for genetic makeup and to market BiDil to the population—namely, African Americans—that appeared to benefit most from the drug. This argument is clearly based on the idea that self-identified race correlates roughly with continental ancestry, which in turn correlates with genetic difference. By contending that race could be used as a proxy for genetic variation, Nissen essentially suggested that on some level African Americans are genetically distinct from other populations. Indeed, he basically geneticized blacks and constructed race as a meaningful biological, genetic category.

BiDil and Its Critics

The geneticization of African Americans through BiDil has been heavily critiqued by a number of social scientists and medical scholars (Hoffman 2005, Kahn 2005, 2013, Bibbins-Domingo and Fernandez 2007, Ellison et al. 2008, Obasogie 2009, Roberts 2011a, 2011b). Their critique centers on the reification of race as a biological, genetic category. The contention is that supporters of BiDil have given race a misplaced concreteness, treating it as an immutable, biological division of humankind rather than as a malleable, socially constructed category. The existence of a drug that is targeted just to African Americans is thus seen as legitimating the idea that races are natural, biological entities—that blacks have particular, intrinsic genetic attributes that function to differentiate them from other groups.

The critique of the genetic reification of race essentially has two strands. One strand focuses on undermining the idea that race (whether self-identified or ascribed) is a genetically meaningful category. For critics, the clearest indication that race is not genetic but rather social in nature is its historical instability: the fact that in the United States racial categories have changed repeatedly over the course of its history. To highlight the instability of race, critics have turned to the US Census. For example, Dorothy Roberts (2011b), one of the leading detractors of BiDil, underscores that every US census has classified people by race, but the racial groupings and their makeup have shifted time and again. She notes:

> The very first US census … in 1790 counted the number of persons in each household according to the following categories: free white males sixteen years and older, free white males under sixteen years, free white females, all other

> free persons, and slaves. ... In the second census, taken in 1800, Indians were specified as a separate category of free persons. Chinese were added to the 1870 census. In 1920, race had become even more complicated. That census included ten racial categories: white, black, mulatto, Indian, Chinese, Japanese, Filipino, Hindu, Korean, and other. By the end of the twentieth century, the racial groupings were consolidated into five main choices: American Indian or Alaska native, Asian, black or African American, native Hawaiian or other Pacific Islander, and white. [Roberts 2011b: 20]

Given this history, Roberts asks rhetorically, "If races are fixed biological groupings, how can the test defining who belongs in each group change? If a person's race is inscribed in her genes, how can a judge officially assign (and reassign) it according to a legal classification system?" (2011b: 20). For Roberts, then, the protean nature of racial groups in the United States is an indication that race is an artifact of state classificatory systems. Indeed, for her, race is basically a political category that reflects social convention, not biology.

Critics have additionally sought to challenge the idea that race is a genetically meaningful category by unraveling the purported link between race and disease or drug response. Consider, for example, the link between African Americans and heart failure. As Jonathan Kahn (2005), another prominent critic of BiDil, has pointed out, NitroMed and other proponents of the drug have stated on numerous occasions that African Americans die from heart failure at twice the rate of whites. This 2:1 mortality statistic was used to support assertions that heart failure represents a different disease in African Americans, and to make the case for a race-specific, genetic approach to treating the condition. It turns out, however, that the 2:1 figure was, according to Kahn, "egregiously wrong" (2005: 116). The rate is actually closer to 1.1:1. The mistaken 2:1 claim came about through a series of miscitations of mortality data from the early 1980s. From Kahn's perspective, then, there is really no difference in heart failure death rates between blacks and whites and thus no justification for regarding heart failure in African Americans as a different disease. Consider also the link between African Americans and the efficacy of heart failure medications. Critics of BiDil have argued that A-HeFT, the trial on which the FDA based its approval of the drug, does not support the idea of racial specificity in drug response (Kahn 2005, Bibbins-Domingo and Fernandez 2007, Obasogie 2009, Roberts 2011b). Their argument is that because A-HeFT enrolled only African Americans (and thus had no comparison population), the trial cannot legitimately be used to assert that BiDil works differently in African Americans. According to Kahn, "the only responsible scientific claim that can be made on the basis of these trials is that BiDil works in some people who have heart failure, period" (2005: 106). For BiDil's critics, there is thus no evidence indicating that BiDil is a pharmocogenetic drug that is differentially efficacious across different racial populations.[4]

The second strand of the critique of racial reification highlights the potentially pernicious consequences of linking race and genetics. Critics of BiDil deem this linking problematic for two main reasons. First of all, given the history of racism in the United States, the geneticization of racialized populations is perceived as having the potential to result in stigmatization and discrimination. Of particular concern is the scientific tendency to associate racial groups with particular disease conditions (for example, African Americans and heart failure). The problems with such association are perhaps most clearly articulated by law professor Sharona Hoffman:

> Public perception that scientific evidence has established that a particular "race" is more vulnerable to life-threatening illnesses than others or does not respond to medications that cure most patients may reinforce negative "race-based" stereotypes and misconceptions. Particular populations may be seen as diseased or incurable. This could fuel the belief that there are inferior human subspecies or biological differences among "races." [Hoffman 2005: 421]

Hoffman further suggests that such stigmatization in turn has the potential to lead to a host of discriminatory practices. As she puts it,

> Some employers may seek to avoid hiring or promoting members of certain "races" because of a fear that they are at high risk of suffering from life-threatening diseases (e.g. cancer) or that they will be untreatable with conventional medicine if they are stricken with serious illnesses (e.g. heart disease). Employers will be concerned about excessive absenteeism, low productivity, and high insurance costs due to above-average medical expenses. [Hoffman 2005: 422]

A prime example Hoffman gives to support the claim of possible stigmatization and discrimination is the association of African Americans with sickle cell anemia (SCA) (see also Roberts 2011b, Kahn 2013). In the United States, the tendency has been to see SCA as a black genetic disease. Hoffman explains that notions about African American susceptibility to SCA have been used to justify the screening of this population for the disease and their exclusion from certain types of employment. In the late 1960s, for example, four black men died while performing combat exercises at a US Army boot camp. The high

4 Critics of BiDil also point out that new research indicates that ACE inhibitors, when taken in combination with diuretics, work just as well in black individuals as in whites. This research thus further counters the idea of racial specificity in drug response (Ellison et al. 2008).

altitude of the camp (over 4,000 feet) and the fact that the red blood cells of the recruits were severely sickled (as revealed by autopsies) were interpreted as indicating that the deaths could have been due to sickle cell crises brought on by the low-oxygen environment. However, a connection between SCA and the death of the recruits was never actually confirmed. Nonetheless, the presumed risk of blood sickling at high altitudes was used to justify denying all black sickle cell carriers—basically healthy individuals who did not in fact have the disease but simply carried one copy of the sickle cell gene—entry into the US Air Force Academy and barring them from serving as commercial airline pilots. Ultimately, these bans were dropped because there was simply no scientific evidence to justify the policies.

The other main reason that critics of BiDil deem the conflation of race and genetics problematic has to do with health disparities. The general claim is that focusing too much on genetics as a root of health disparities and emphasizing race-targeted pharmacology as a solution to such inequities unnecessarily takes attention away from the social determinants of disease (Kahn 2003, Brody and Hunt 2006, Bibbins-Domingo and Fernandez 2007, Roberts 2011a). For instance, Dorothy Roberts suggests that because NitroMed researchers chose to focus their research (as exemplified by the GRAHF study) on finding genetic mechanisms to explain BiDil's efficacy, they in effect discounted environmental causes. As she puts it, "By leaping to a genetic explanation, [researchers] foreclosed a potentially more fruitful investigation of the environmental factors that separate white and black health—and that could improve prevention of heart disease for everyone" (Roberts 2011a: 18). Ultimately, the issue for critics is that the framing of health disparities as a genetic matter might lead to a misallocation of health care resources. Jonathan Kahn articulates this concern as follows:

> To the extent that there are real health disparities that correlate with racial groups, an over-emphasis on genetics as an explanation for the disparity can lead to a misallocation of intellectual and material resources. For example, hypertension (a primary cause of heart failure) is caused by a wide array of factors, some social and environmental, some genetic. There are disparities in the incidence of hypertension between blacks and whites. The drive to reduce such racial disparities to a function of genetic variation fuels a logic that would concentrate resources needed to redress disparities on pharmaceutical interventions that work at the molecular level, rather than addressing large issues of diet, behavior, racism, and economic inequity that also play significant roles in hypertension. [Kahn 2003: 479]

For BiDil's critics, then, the practice of geneticizing African Americans may hamper the effort to address the problem of health disparities.

Enlightened Geneticization of Race

The fears raised about BiDil are unquestionably serious. There is no doubt that the geneticization of African Americans can open the door to discriminatory treatment and lead to the reproduction of health disparities. However, critics of BiDil have not done justice to the complexities of how NitroMed and other supporters of the drug have geneticized (or not) African Americans. Contrary to the way BiDil's advocates have been portrayed, they do not necessarily, or at least not explicitly, reify race, nor are they generally determinists who reduce the causes of intricate biological and social processes to genetics. Their geneticization of African Americans can generally be best characterized as enlightened: a nonreductionist, nonessentialist type of geneticization that presents a complex view of race and illness, acknowledges the importance of both genetic and nongenetic factors in disease causation, and does not construct "races" as discrete genetic entities. Indeed, it is clear that most BiDil advocates are cognizant that race is a rather vague indicator of genetic difference and that health inequities cannot be reduced to genes.

We can elaborate on the enlightened geneticization of race by looking first at the question of health disparities. It is certainly the case that NitroMed has suggested a genetic basis for heart failure among blacks, but the company has not ignored social and environmental causes. On their Heart.Health.Heritage website, in response to the question, "Why are African Americans at greater risk?" NitroMed answered, "African Americans are at a much higher risk for heart failure in part because more of them develop high blood pressure and diabetes than other ethnic groups" (NitroMed 2006a). The company further notes that other likely causes of heart failure include poor access to good health care services, greater exposure to environmental pollutants, and a propensity to be overweight and to exercise less. NitroMed thus recommends "accessing better health care, getting regular checkups, eating right, and staying active" to help prevent heart disease (ABC and NitroMed n.d.). Keith Ferdinand likewise points to the importance of social determinants in heart failure, suggesting that "the factors of socioeconomic status, sodium intake, obesity, and physical inactivity may have profound effects on the prevalence and severity of hypertension, HF, and other cardiovascular conditions" (Ferdinand 2006b: 158). Thus, although Ferdinand advocates that researchers continue to "measure the effects of the genetic influence on cardiovascular diseases," he also exhorts clinicians to "utilize clinical judgment and assist patients with understanding the importance of lifestyle modifications" (2006b: 158).

With regard to the construction of race as a genetic category, NitroMed and ABC scientists do suggest that blacks may be more genetically prone to developing heart failure, but this is not the same as saying that races exist as clearly differentiated genetic entities or even that they exist at all biologically.

In fact, supporters of BiDil have generally emphasized that race is a social category. Clyde Yancy articulates this perspective most forcefully:

> Race is neither physiologic nor scientific; rather it is a social construct that reflects a group of persons with shared ancestry and similar customs/lifestyles that also intermarry. Clearly, African Americans represent a heterogeneous group and there is no reason to believe that any single genetic trait is uniformly and exclusively distributed in African Americans. Race is not a proxy for genetics and any effort to ascribe such is shallow and lacking understanding. However, within this group, it is conceivable that certain traits may be over represented and that these traits might contribute to disease. [2007]

NitroMed and the ABC also emphasize that the indication of BiDil for blacks only does not mean that the drug will not work on other populations (Cohn 2003: S209, Ferdinand 2006b: 158). On the basis of the GRAHF substudy, NitroMed in fact argues that the genetic markers that may predict a patient's response to BiDil "are not unique to any one racial group—although they may be more prevalent in one group versus another" (NitroMed 2007d). The geneticization of African Americans thus does not necessarily amount to a reification of race. Indeed, when NitroMed and the ABC connect race to genetics, they do so not with the aim of objectifying racial groups as genetic entities—as homogeneous, immutable biological divisions among humankind. Rather, their goal is simply to understand how genetics might help account for differences in disease incidence and drug response between socially constructed human populations.

It should also be noted that some strong supporters of BiDil do not resort to the geneticization of African Americans. For them, the explanation of black health disparities lies in the social experiences of this population. Indeed, their concern has been with race as a social phenomenon with bodily consequences, rather than as a genetic or biological category. The views of Congresswoman Donna Christensen can serve as an illustration. In her remarks before the FDA's Cardiovascular and Renal Drugs Advisory Committee, Christensen argued that, genetically speaking, humans are essentially all alike. She stated, "We know that all of us no matter the color of our skin, or race or ethnic origin are 99% the same genetically" (Christensen 2005: 207). For her, the existence of BiDil does not change this fact. Crucially, Christensen also makes the suggestion that the category "black" should be interpreted as including "all of the 'social' forces and biological feedback loops that Dr. Troy Duster admonishes us to understand" (2005: 208). The reference to Troy Duster is key. A noted sociologist of race and science, Duster has argued that "race and racial categories can best be understood as a set of social processes that can create biological consequences; race is a set of social processes with biological feedbacks that require empirical investigation" (Ossorio and Duster 2005: 116). The idea here is simply that the experience of race has an effect on the biological functioning of the body. An example that Duster (2007) gives is hypertension. He notes that in the United States African Americans with darker skin tend to have higher rates of the disease. Scientists have persistently attempted to link this connection between hypertension and skin color to genetics. Duster suggests, however, that the higher rates of hypertension among darker skinned blacks are due not to genetics but to the fact that having darker skin subjects people to greater discrimination. He articulates this stance as follows: "the correlation between skin color and hypertension [is] not biological or genetic in origin, but biological in effect due to stress-related outcomes of reduced access to valued social goods, such as employment, promotion, housing stock, etc." (Duster 2007: 703). Returning to Congresswoman Christensen, the point is that she understands the diseases that befall African Americans as the biological materializations of social inequality. Her concern is not with genetics but with "the many social, political and economic variants which define being an African American in the United States today" (Christensen 2005: 208).

Although NitroMed and other BiDil advocates are aware that the relationship between race and genetics is quite complex, their enlightened geneticization of race nevertheless has problematic elements. One problem is that, in supporting BiDil as a racially specific drug, advocates end up implicitly endorsing a model of genetic difference that reifies race. Essentially, the FDA's approval of BiDil for blacks only gives the impression, even if not intended, that African Americans constitute a discrete genetic grouping: that they have inherent genetic characteristics that serve to demarcate them from other racialized populations. Indeed, it would not make sense to approve the drug for just African Americans unless there was something genetically specific about this population. However, there is nothing genetically unique about African Americans to warrant the existence of a drug just for them. BiDil's critics have of course pointed out that the historical instability of racial categories in the United States demonstrates that "races" are social and not genetic in nature. But even if we were to grant that race, as understood in the United States, could be used as a proxy for genetic difference, this does not mean that racial groups can be clearly distinguished from one another. Human genetic variation does not work that way. As geneticists Rick Kittles and Kenneth Weiss explain,

> human genetic variation is actually characterized by clines (spatial gradients) of allele frequency rather than categorical variation between populations, and the pattern varies among genes for the historic reasons of drift, selection, and demographic history. Even defined in the usual ways, races do not correspond to discrete, much less monomorphic, human types. Instead, the pattern of variation can generally be described as isolation by distance: Genetic differences

> between populations are roughly proportional to the geographic distance between them. [2003: 37–8]

The point here is that because genetic variation is continuous, it is impossible to draw a line that clearly separates one racial group from another (Goodman, Moses, and Jones 2012). To designate a drug for African Americans alone, treating this population as if it were a distinct genetic entity, is thus very much a fallacy.

A second problem is that NitroMed and other BiDil advocates also implicitly endorse a model of pharmaceutical development that appears to ignore both intragroup variability and overlap across groups in drug response. In addition to giving the impression that blacks are a unique genetic entity, the FDA's approval of BiDil only for African Americans seemingly suggests that the drug will work on all blacks. This is simply not the case, however. It is commonly accepted among population geneticists that the vast majority—approximately 85 percent—of human genetic variation is within-group variation (Ossorio and Duster 2005). Unrelated individuals of the same racial group are thus not particularly similar to each other genetically. Indeed, any racial group is genetically quite heterogeneous. Given that African Americans are a genetically diverse population, any drug, including BiDil, will work on some members and not on others. The approval of BiDil thus appears to ignore the fact that individuals of the same racial group vary in how they respond to drugs (Root 2003: 1178). It is also the case that even if there are differences between how various populations react to drugs, they all tend to overlap significantly in their response. Summarizing a paper (Sehgal 2004) that analyzes data from 15 studies of antihypertensive drugs, Steven Epstein (2007: 220) notes that "even though whites on average responded better to beta-blockers and ACE inhibitors than blacks did, and blacks on average responded better to diuretics and calcium-channel blockers than whites did, overall 80 to 95 percent of blacks and whites had similar responses to these various drugs." The implication here is that there is little scientific justification for approving a drug for just one population.

A final problem has to do with race and health disparities. It is clear that NitroMed and other BiDil supporters generally make room for environmental factors in disease causality and do not reduce disorders to genes. However, their support of genetics as a way of dealing with health disparities, even if not reductionist, is problematic. Critics of BiDil have correctly pointed out that too much attention to genetics in disease causality might divert attention away from the social determinants of disease and lead to the reproduction of health inequalities (Kahn 2003, Roberts 2011a). The basic problem is that investing in genetic research is not necessarily the most productive way to address the issue of health disparities (Sankar 2006), because genetics cannot generally account for racial health disparities. For example, there is no doubt that African

Americans tend to suffer disproportionately from a host of maladies, ranging from diabetes and hypertension to breast and prostate cancers. But it is not the case that these health disparities can be attributed principally to genetic factors (Sankar et al. 2004).[5] If genetics had a strong influence on the health status of African Americans, one would expect that African-origin populations around the world would experience similar health outcomes. Instead, research generally shows that blacks living outside the United States suffer from the maladies just noted at far lower rates (Cooper 2004, Sankar et al. 2004). This is not to say that genetics plays no role in explaining health disparities, but this role is likely to be rather small. As bioethicist Pamela Sankar (2006) has pointed out, genetic mutations that cause disease are rather unusual and not typically implicated in most occurrences of common illnesses. Using a specific disease as an example, she explains:

> [P]rostate cancer among black men is often cited as one of the potentially most useful targets for genetic research. Between 1995 and 2000, statistics show that there were 73 prostate cancer deaths per 100,000 black men and only 30 per 100,000 white men. Approximately 10% to 15% of prostate cancer deaths are believed to have hereditary causes. ... If scientists discovered the genes for prostate cancer risk among black men tomorrow, and discovered a way to use this information to eliminate the morbidity due to genetic prostate cancer (the latter being far more difficult than the former), the number of prostate cancer deaths per year per 100,000 black men would decrease by 7 to 10 cases, to approximately 63 to 66 per 100,000, a rate still more than double that of white men, thus still leaving in place a large unexplained imbalance. [Sankar 2006: 254]

After genetics is taken into consideration, then, most of the disparity in African American prostate cancer rates remains to be explained.

Although genetics cannot generally account for racial disparities in health, social and environmental factors can. Indeed, a plethora of scientific research points to the importance of the social environment in determining the health outcomes of racial minority populations in the United States (Frank 2001, Sankar et al. 2004, Krieger 2005, Shields et al. 2005, Brooks and King 2008). Key social factors that contribute to health disparities include persistent racial discrimination and lack of access to (or inferior) medical treatment (Smedley, Stith, and Nelson

5 The linking of health disparities to genetics points to another problem: the potential for racial inferiorization. Given that minority populations are disproportionately afflicted with a range of illnesses, any research or policy that associates their poor health with genetic predisposition to disease could be interpreted as suggesting that these racial groups are naturally biologically inferior to groups who experience better health outcomes (Sankar et al. 2004).

2003, Sankar 2006). For example, pervasive and enduring racial discrimination has produced patterns of residential segregation that confine minorities to inferior housing and neighborhoods (Sankar 2006). In these surroundings, groups such as African Americans and Latinos are likely to be exposed to a host of health hazards, including toxic chemicals, lead paint, air pollution, unsafe wiring, allergens produced by rodent and insect infestations, and so forth. Furthermore, racial discrimination has had the effect of relegating minorities to substandard schools and low-wage jobs (Williams and Collins 2001, Sankar 2006). The resulting poverty, and the fact that low-paying jobs do not generally offer health insurance, make it difficult for racial minority populations to have access to health care (Brooks and King 2008). And when they do have access, it is often to community health clinics and public hospitals that tend to provide poorer quality care. Taken together, social factors such as unsafe living conditions and inadequate health care lead to shorter and less healthy lives for racial minority populations, particularly blacks, Latinos, and Native Americans (Sankar 2006). Increasing access to quality care and improving the living conditions of minorities is thus likely to be more productive than investing in genetic research.

Conclusion

I have argued in this chapter that proponents of BiDil—whether the FDA, NitroMed, or African Americans themselves—do not generally advocate any kind of crude genetic reductionism. For example, in regard to health disparities, NitroMed has certainly suggested a genetic basis for heart failure among blacks, but the company has not ignored social and environmental causes. Regarding the construction of race as a biological category, NitroMed and its scientists may argue that blacks may be more genetically prone to developing heart failure, but this is not the same as saying that races exist as homogeneous, clearly differentiated genetic entities. At the same time, it is also clear that BiDil is not problem free. Scientifically, a wealth of evidence suggests that while there may be differences in how populations react to drugs, overall they tend to overlap significantly in their response. There is thus no reason to target drugs to specific populations. And politically, even though supporters of BiDil take social factors into account in the etiology of disease, their promotion of genetics as a way to solve the problem of health disparities supports a line of research that is not likely to reduce health disparities and could even reproduce them. What all this suggests is that "race" needs to be treated not as a genetic category but as a social one. Indeed, it is clear that racial categories are very much socio-political constructs (Lee at al. 2008, Roberts 2011b). The solution to the problem of health disparities thus lies not in genetic research but in improving the social conditions of minority populations.

Chapter 5
Racial Vital Value

In the previous chapter, I focused on BiDil and its problematic geneticization of race. This is not the drug's only issue, however. Also problematic is the use of BiDil in efforts to capitalize on racial life. On the whole, the cultivation of life and health in the United States has come to be intimately linked to the production of wealth (Rose 2007). Without question, biomedicine and the biosciences today are highly subject to the exigencies of capitalization, with shareholder demands and profit obligations heavily shaping the medical problems that these knowledges of life seek to address. Pharmaceutical companies have been key players in this capitalization of life. Though the manufacture of pharmaceuticals, they have sought not only to enhance the vitality of life and the body, but also, just as importantly, to generate economic profits. In this context, racial life has emerged as a potential source of value, or what might be called *racial vital value*: the economic value generated by fostering the vitality of racial bodies.

In this chapter, I look at BiDil and the economic valuation of racial life. There is no doubt that commercial factors have been a driving force behind the production of the drug as a racial pharmaceutical. As noted in Chapter 2, the scientists who developed BiDil first sought to have the drug approved for the general population. When the FDA turned them down, they went back to the data from their initial clinical trials (the Veterans Affairs Vasodilator-Heart Failure Trials, V-HeFT I and II), reanalyzed it along racial lines, and concluded that BiDil appeared to work better in blacks than in whites. Race thus came to matter only following the FDA's rejection. The BiDil scientists essentially turned to race to salvage the drug. They were able to do this in part because of the propitious political climate. The reanalysis of the BiDil data took place in the context of increasing political desire to address race and gender disparities in health care. The scientists were also able to turn to race because African Americans have a socio-political identity that makes them a powerful market force. Indeed, as health sciences scholar George Ellison has pointed out, "it's possible to develop a drug for African Americans because we can identify them, we can market to them, we can sell it to them" (Malik 2005). On some level, then, BiDil's production as a racial medication appears to have been not simply about saving African American lives but also about the profits to be derived from saving the drug itself.

Economization of Life

The advent of BiDil, and its relation to questions of racial vital value, is best understood in the context of transformations in global capitalism and the emergence of what has come to be called the *bioeconomy* (OECD 2006, Rose 2007). According to David Harvey, the worldwide depression of 1973–75 signaled a major change in the development of capitalism:

> The twenty-year postwar boom that preceded [the depression] produced strong growth rates (over 4.4 percent per year), relatively low unemployment, relatively controlled inflation, and stable exchange rates and commodity prices in most of the advanced capitalist world. ... US hegemony and the clear-cut geopolitics of the Cold War anchored this postwar capitalist world militarily, economically, and politically. After the 1973–75 depression, capitalist economies entered a period of difficult readjustment and restructuring, sparked by low growth rates (roughly 2.2 percent per year from 1973 to 1988), high unemployment and inflation, and the breakdown of US hegemony. [1991: 66–7]

Put otherwise, the countries of the advanced capitalist world generally suffered through a "crisis of Fordism" in the late twentieth century (Harrison and Bluestone 1988, Calavita 1996). From World War II to the mid-1970s, these countries operated (rather profitably) on Fordist principles of mass production, an economic formation centered on standardized products for mass consumption, vertically integrated firms with internal job ladders, relative employment security, Keynesian economic policy, and state protection of national economies from the vagaries of capitalism (Calavita 1996, Gottweis, Salter, and Waldby 2009). Beginning in the 1970s, however, the Fordist system began to unravel as line-balancing issues (that is, shortages and gluts in production inputs and inventory), a generally inflexible structure of production, corporate taxation policies, and labor strife coalesced to undermine corporate profitability (Calavita 1996). In the United States, for example, the average profit rate of nonfinancial corporations dropped from 10 percent in 1965 to slightly more than 5 percent in the late 1970s (Harrison and Bluestone 1988). As the Fordist regime collapsed, a new economic structure emerged as companies seeking to retool turned to novel sources of profitability in the form of more flexible forms of production and technological innovation (Gottweis, Salter, and Waldby 2009). This post-Fordist system is characterized by "just-in-time" production strategies, labor cost reductions (through contingent and part-time work arrangements), flexibility in hiring and firing, the development of niche markets, the general retrenchment of the welfare state, and crucially, an emphasis on the commercial exploitation of scientific knowledge (Harvey 1989, Calavita 1998).

One key area of scientific knowledge that has been tapped as a source of potential profit, particularly in the United States, is the life sciences. Indeed, the biosciences, including biomedicine, have come to be highly integrated into market regimes (Cooper 2008, Sunder Rajan 2006, 2007, 2012a).[1] The "corporatization of the life sciences" can be traced to the 1970s with the advent of recombinant DNA technology (RDT) and the concomitant birth of the biotech industry (Sunder Rajan 2012a). RDT, a molecular technique for isolating and combining fragments of DNA, revolutionized the life sciences by making it possible not only to know genes better but also to manipulate them in ways useful for the development of commercial applications in medicine, agriculture, forensics, veterinary medicine, and environmental pollution.[2] Subsequent to the invention of RDT, a host of changes during the 1980s in the legal and regulatory structures governing bio-innovations significantly opened up the life sciences to capitalization. Specifically, the Bayh-Dole Act (1980), which enabled the transfer of technology between universities and industry in the United States, facilitated the commercialization of basic research, while the US Supreme Court ruling *Diamond v Chakrabarty* (1980), which permitted patent rights on a genetically engineered microorganism, enabled the patenting of life forms. Given the potential profitability of the life sciences, commercial enterprises seeking to reorganize after the decline of Fordist industrial production came to invest large amounts of venture capital in university-based research, biotech companies, pharmaceutical ventures, and so forth (Gottweis, Salter, and Waldby 2009). Ultimately, this large-scale capitalization of the biosciences would give rise to what has come to be called the *bioeconomy*, a sphere of economic activity that encompasses the totality of research and innovation in the biological sciences (OECD 2006, Rose 2007, White House 2012). Today, the bioeconomy—responsible for such innovations as the mapping of the human genome, stem cell technologies, protein engineering, cloning, and nanotechnology—is a significant and ever growing sector of the world economy.

There are two important aspects of the bioeconomy that I want to highlight. First, in the bioeconomy, life is a central locus of value (Sunder Rajan 2006, Rose 2007), in particular of what I will call *vital value*.[3] Vital value refers to how the vitality of individuals and populations functions as a potential source of

1 Kaushik Sunder Rajan (2007: 80) uses the term *biocapital* to capture how the life sciences have come to be imbricated in "frameworks of capital and the market," while Melinda Cooper (2008) explores the rise of the life sciences alongside neoliberal economics.

2 Commercial applications include gene therapy, the molecular diagnosis of diseases, DNA fingerprinting, genetically modified foods, vaccines, and pharmaceutical products.

3 For a different articulation of the term *vital value*, see Mol 1998.

profitability.[4] The idea here is simply that the life sciences, especially biomedicine, derive economic value from cultivating the vitality of the human body. Vital value is generated through the exploitation of individuals and populations as therapeutic markets.[5] As anthropologist Kaushik Sunder Rajan has noted,

> In biomedicine, the materialization of value occurs through the production of treatments. A patient is valuable to biomedicine to the extent that she takes treatments and continues to take them—a healthy patient who is not on, or is not likely to be on, medication is, from the perspective of this economy, not valuable. [2012b: 328]

Essentially, what the biosciences generally do is take the body's cellular or molecular fragments—DNA, stem cells, oöcytes, and so forth—and work to instrumentalize them in ways that can lead to the development of commercial technologies designed to nurture the vitality of the living (Waldby 2000, 2002, Rose 2007). The knowledge created by the biological sciences is thus expected to produce not just truths about the body but also marketable goods (that is, therapeutic or clinical applications) that can be deployed to safeguard and improve bodily health. Indeed, as Paul Rabinow has pointed out,

> More than ever before, the legitimacy of the life sciences now rests on claims to produce health. Having tilted too heavily in the direction of quasi utilitarian ends … the bioscience community now runs the risk that merely producing truth will be insufficient to move the venture capitalists, patent offices, and science writers on whom the biosciences are increasingly dependent for their new-found wealth. [1996: 137]

Vital value, then, is at once about vitality and profitability. It involves both the enhancement of human health and the creation of economic wealth. Vital

---

4 My term *vital value* is similar to Catherine Waldby's notion of *biovalue*, which she defines as "the yield of vitality produced by the biotechnical reformulation of living processes" (Waldby 2002: 310). Her concept emphasizes how value is extracted from living processes by way of technical manipulation. By contrast, in *vital value* it is vitality itself that is the potential source of value. The stress is less on the manipulation of living processes and more on the economic value that can be derived from fostering the vitality of the body.

5 The life sciences also exploit individuals and populations as biological resources. However, the use of the body as a resource does not in and of itself yield vital value. Vital value is generated only at the point of consumption, when therapeutic and clinical applications (which may be derived from the body) reach their markets and enhance the vitality of the living.

value is produced when therapeutic products simultaneously generate profits and foster the health and vitality of individuals and populations.

The second important aspect of the bioeconomy that I want to highlight is niche marketing. Accounts of the transition from Fordism to post-Fordism have emphasized that the practice of producing mass products for mass markets has generally given way to the practice of producing custom-tailored goods for specialized markets (Amin 1994). Niche marketing has made especially significant inroads into biomedicine (Epstein 2007, Clarke et al. 2010). Although one-size-fits-all medical devices, technologies, and drugs continue to be the norm in the medical field, the customization of such products on the basis of race, age, sex, and gender has become increasingly common. Important cases of biomedical customization can be found in the pharmaceutical industry, where drug companies have gradually developed more medications for specific populations. For instance, women have become distinctive targets of pharmaceutical intervention. Some medications produced for women are for conditions specific to them. Examples of such drugs are the contraceptive pill and hormone replacement therapy (used to relieve the symptoms of menopause). Other medications developed for women are for conditions that are believed to affect women and men differently (cancer and heart disease, for instance). Examples of such medications are Zelnorm and Lotronex, both of which treat irritable bowl syndrome. In 2002, they became the first drugs endorsed by the FDA for just women to treat a malady that afflicts both sexes (Epstein 2007). Men too have become valuable targets of pharmaceutical intervention. The most well-known drug developed for men is Viagra (Clarke et al. 2010), which treats erectile dysfunction, but there are also others, including Rogaine (for hair loss), Zytiga (for prostate cancer), and Flomax (for the symptoms of an enlarged prostate). Finally, racial groups have also become targets of pharmaceutical niche marketing. The premier example of a racially-marketed drug is clearly BiDil. However, as we will see, BiDil is not the only drug being marketed to specific racial groups. Also important are Travatan, used to treat intraocular pressure, and Bystolic, an antihypertensive. Both drugs have been touted as effective in treating African Americans (Roberts 2011b, Kahn 2013).

BiDil, Vital Value, and Niche Marketing

BiDil is intimately concerned with both the creation of vital value and the exploitation of niche markets. More precisely, the drug is involved in the production of *racial vital value* because the generation of profits is tied to fostering the vitality of the racial body, and it is implicated in the exploitation of racial niche markets because the target market is a racialized population:

African Americans. With respect to producing racial vital value, there is no doubt that BiDil is concerned with cultivating the vitality of living racial beings. As discussed in Chapter 3, the drug has been promoted as a life-saving and life-improving technology. On an individual level, BiDil promises to save African American lives and improve the quality of a person's everyday living. The mere existence of the drug makes the statement that the maladies of African Americans are worthy of being remedied and that black lives merit saving. On a collective level, BiDil promises to reduce health disparities. The aspiration is to improve the collective well-being of African Americans by reducing their rates of cardiovascular disease so that they are on par with the rates of other populations. Although it is not likely that BiDil will lead to the amelioration of health inequalities, because it does not deal with the social determinants of heart failure (see Chapter 4), indications are that in some ways the drug does foster racial life: it does save lives and improve the quality of individual existence. The results of the African American Heart Failure Trial (A-HeFT) showed that, in comparison to the placebo group, individuals on BiDil experienced a 43 percent reduction in the risk of mortality and a noticeable improvement in their quality of life (Taylor et al. 2004). BiDil is thus clearly implicated in producing longer and healthier African American lives. The drug is about cultivating racial health and vitality.

It is evident that BiDil is also about profiting from fostering the vitality of the racial body. In fact, it appears that the emergence of BiDil as a racial drug was propelled to a large degree by market incentives (Bloche 2004, Roberts 2011b, Kahn 2013). As mentioned earlier, BiDil did not start out as a race-specific drug. Race became relevant only after the FDA turned down the initial New Drug Application (NDA) for using the medication on the general population. It became relevant basically as a means to save the drug. Dr. Jay Cohn and NitroMed have made clear on a number of occasions that they believe the drug will work on all populations, not just on blacks. For example, in an interview with the *Los Angeles Times* on June 16, 2005, Cohn stated, "I actually think everybody should be using it [BiDil]" (Gellene 2005). He further noted that he prescribed hydralazine hydrochloride and isosorbide dinitrate (H/I), the generic components that make up BiDil, to 25 percent of his white patients for whom other drugs were not effective. Similarly, Dr. Michael Loberg, former president and CEO of NitroMed, has asserted that even though A-HeFT proved the efficacy of BiDil only on African Americans, "[i]t doesn't mean that others won't benefit [from the drug] as well" (Saul 2005a). Given this strong conviction that BiDil would work on all populations, the resort to race can best be explained as a strategic maneuver to salvage the drug. The overriding goal, it appears, was simply to bring the drug to the marketplace, with a race-delimited market being better than no market at all. In addition to allowing BiDil to be rescued, race also permitted the life of the drug's patent to be extended.

This is important because, in the pharmaceutical industry, profits hinge on patents and the market exclusivity they confer (Fisher 2009). By the time the first NDA for BiDil was rejected in 1997, only ten years remained in the patent life of the drug, which was set to expire in 2007 (Sankar and Kahn 2005). So even if Cohn, who created BiDil, had been able to secure the drug's approval for the general population, little patent life, and hence profitability, would have remained. However, by turning to race and obtaining a race-specific patent (see Chapter 2), Cohn significantly extended BiDil's market protection and revenue potential. The race-specific patent gave its owner sole rights to sell the H/I combination to African Americans for 13 years beyond the original patent—until 2020 (Sankar and Kahn 2005). Race, then, essentially gave BiDil's stakeholders an opportunity to extract profits from what otherwise would have been a failed drug (Roberts 2011b, Kahn 2013).

A central reason, it is important to note, why race could be utilized to salvage BiDil was that African Americans constitute a powerful consumer market niche.[6] Indeed, if they were not a potent market force, pharmaceutical companies would not be producing drugs just for them. Racial vital value and racial niche marketing are thus very much intertwined. The key to the commercial success of any pharmacogenetic drug is finding the right market.[7] Because pharmacogenetic medicines target not the general population but rather subgroups with specific genetic profiles, the pool of consumers available to buy such drugs is necessarily limited. As Dorothy Roberts points out, the "challenge is to determine where to draw the line between the subgroups so that they are personalized enough to define drug targets but large enough to guarantee a profit" (2011b: 163). Taking the United States as a market, if the subgroups targeted were too small—say persons of such national origin ancestries as Japanese, Korean, French, Ethiopian, and Mexican—it would be too expensive for pharmaceutical companies to create drugs specifically for them. It appears, however, that racially demarcated minority groups—blacks, Asians, and Latinos—offer large enough patient pools that it can make financial sense to treat those populations as markets for pharmaceutical products. Indeed, there is a strong sense among health care marketing firms that racial markets are potentially profitable. An article in the magazine *Multicultural Health Marketing* put it as follows:

6 Also key, of course, were scientific developments that gave weight to the idea that genetic differences between racially demarcated groups are important in terms of drug response and political efforts to eliminate racial health disparities (see Chapter 2).

7 BiDil is of course not technically a pharmacogenetic drug, because its efficacy has not been linked to specific genes. However, the drug has been billed as a pharmacogenetic medicine because it is believed to have different effects depending on the population.

> The 2011 U.S. Census revealed a startling fact: For the first time, racial and ethnic minorities made up more than half the children born in America. The vast majority—more than a third of the country's entire population—are black and Latino. Those are large numbers, but when chronic diseases are considered, the numbers soar—in a different kind of way. According to the Centers for Disease Control and Prevention, African Americans have the highest age-adjusted death rate for heart disease, cancer, diabetes and HIV/AIDS.
>
> Health marketers and communicators cannot do their job effectively without reaching minority populations. [Bailey and Jones 2012: 14]

Racial markets are potential moneymakers, then, because racialized minorities are increasing in number and have a higher burden of disease than the general population (Roberts 2011b).

Beyond population numbers and disease prevalence rates, it is also the case that minorities, African Americans in particular, have proven purchasing power. In a report on the multicultural economy, the University of Georgia's Selig Center for Economic Growth estimates that black buying power in 2004, just prior to the approval of BiDil, was $723 billion (Humphreys 2004: 3). This figure was up from $318 billion in 1990 and $585 billion in 2000. By 2009, the projected buying power of African Americans was expected to be $965 billion. From 1990 to 2009, then, the percentage change in black purchasing power was forecast to be 203 percent, indicating that African Americans were a large and fast-growing niche market. Indeed, as noted in the report,

> This overall percentage gain outstrips the 140 percent increase in white buying power and the 159 percent increase in total buying power (all races combined). In 2009, the nation's share of total buying power that is black will be 8.7 percent, up from 8.4 percent in 2004 and up from 7.4 percent in 1990. Nationally, African-American consumers will account for almost nine cents out of every dollar that is spent. [Humphreys 2004: 3]

To cater to this large and growing African American consumer market, businesses have established a race-based marketing infrastructure (Roberts 2011b) consisting of advertizing agencies such as Burrell Communications, Footsteps, IMAGES USA, and Walton Isaacson; research companies such as Geoscape, The Hunter-Miller Group, Knowledge Networks, and Millward-Brown; and marketing consultants such as Diversity Affluence and New American Dimensions. The objective of this infrastructure is basically to help brands and businesses understand and market to ethnic consumers. Thus, from sports, media, and music to hair products, shoes, alcohol, and cigarettes, consumer products are routinely marketed by race.

For NitroMed, then, African Americans represented a ready-made and potentially lucrative market for BiDil. Not only did this community have buying power, but they also had perceived unmet medical needs that could be targeted as a way to make profits. Speaking at a webcast presentation announcing the launch of BiDil, Michael Loberg noted:

> We know that the market potential here is actually at the high end of what we might have expected based on the package insert. The drug extends life. It enhances patient reported functional status. ... It reduces cost that saves the payor's money. And there is a large unmet need for this drug in an overburdened, underserved population. It is in some cases the marketer's dream. [NitroMed 2005e]

As part of the same webcast, Mark Pavao, senior vice president of sales and marketing, put a dollar figure on the market value of African American heart failure sufferers: "The black heart failure marketplace ... is also a very significant marketplace, approximately 750,000 black heart failure patients, classes II to IV. And that by itself ... at the BiDil pricing leads to a potential market opportunity over a billion dollars" (NitroMed 2005e). The billion-dollar amount was a bit of an exaggeration, as Pavao himself acknowledged. To reach it would require that all black heart failure patients take BiDil. However, the potential market value of the drug was still considerable. In 2004, Liana Moussatos, an analyst for Pacific Growth Equities, estimated that BiDil could deliver sales of about $350 million by 2010 (Kennedy 2004). This number was subsequently adjusted in 2005 to between $450 and $500 million after NitroMed announced the pricing of the drug at $1.80 per pill (Saul 2005b). Other analysts—namely the Friedman, Billings, Ramsey Group, an investment bank—put the potential sales of the drug at around $825 million annually (Saul 2005a).

To help sell BiDil to African Americans, NitroMed tapped into the infrastructure of racial niche marketing. In 2004, in anticipation of the drug's approval, NitroMed hired Vigilante, a black-led advertising agency, to provide creative support for its marketing campaign (Holmes 2004, Roberts 2011b, Kahn 2013). In announcing the deal, B.J. Jones, vice president of marketing for NitroMed, stated, "Vigilante maintains a highly regarded reputation and continues to remain a leader in the field of advertising and marketing to the African American, minority, and urban communities. We welcome Vigilante's years of expertise to support NitroMed's commercialization of BiDil in the coming months" (Holmes 2004). Vigilante's customers have included Heineken, Western Union, General Motors, Nike, and the United States Tennis Association (Thomaselli 2005, Rusert and Royal 2011). The agency also worked with the *Oprah Winfrey Show* to publicize its now famous giveaway of Pontiac G-6 sports sedans to the audience at the 19th season premiere. One of the principal aims of the campaign developed by Vigilante was to educate black consumers about BiDil. As Vigilante's president and chief executive officer Larry Woodard noted, "education will be a focal point of the campaign as it aims to increase awareness about the drug" (Holmes 2004). The hope was that by arming African American heart failure sufferers with knowledge about the benefits of BiDil, this population would then ask their doctors to prescribe the medication. With this educational goal in mind, Vigilante's advertising campaign principally entailed running radio spots and print ads (in black newspapers) about BiDil in cities with large African American populations, such as Detroit, Houston, and Washington, DC. Vigilante and NitroMed also placed ads in the national black magazine *Jet*.[8]

BiDil's Failure

Clearly there were high hopes that BiDil would be profitable. Indeed, the expectation was that the drug would generate significant vital value. As it turns out, however, BiDil has been a market failure. On January 15, 2008, NitroMed announced that it was halting the marketing of the drug (NitroMed 2008a).[9] The company stated that although sales of BiDil had been increasing, it did not have enough resources to mount the "marketing and sales effort" necessary for the drug "to achieve its full potential" (NitroMed 2008a). The reality is that from the outset sales of BiDil were low. Analysts had estimated that revenue from the drug would total $130 million in 2006 (Westphal 2006). That year, however, BiDil made only $12.1 million (Westphal 2006). The next year, 2007, sales of the drug were only marginally better, totaling a mere $15.3 million (NitroMed 2008b). Ultimately, NitroMed was not able to survive as a standalone entity. On January 27, 2009, the company announced that it had agreed to be acquired by Deerfield Management, an investment company focused on health care (NitroMed 2009). Deerfield then turned around and sold NitroMed to Arbor Pharmaceuticals in December 2011 (Elsevier Business Intelligence 2011). The new company has resumed marketing BiDil and plans to conduct research, as

8 Hiring Vigilante was only part of NitroMed's overall marketing strategy. The company also developed a grassroots campaign that involved working with African American organizations (churches, the NAACP, and so forth) to get the word about BiDil out to black consumers (Jewell 2006). NitroMed's marketing targets were not just black heart failure sufferers, but also the primary care physicians, cardiologists, and other caregivers who treated this population. To reach these caregivers, NitroMed hired a workforce of 195 sales representatives (NitroMed 2005e).

9 Although NitroMed discontinued its sales and promotional activities for BiDil, the company kept the drug on the market and available for patients.

one company spokesperson put it, "to try to predict more accurately which patients are most likely to respond to the treatment" (Downey 2012: 1876). It remains to be seen if BiDil will experience a successful rebirth and achieve its commercial promise.

BiDil's market failure is a remarkable development for a drug invested with so much financial promise. Besides NitroMed's lack of adequate capital to market the drug, a number of reasons can be offered for BiDil's disappointing commercial life. Prominent among these reasons is the high cost of the drug. At $1.80 per pill, BiDil was priced considerably higher than its generic alternatives (Séguin et al. 2008: 171). With patients having to take the drug three times a day, at either one or two pills per dose, the cost of BiDil came to around $5.40 to $10.80 per day. Given this high cost and the availability of cheaper generics, NitroMed had a tough time getting BiDil included in a number of major health insurance plans (Séguin et al. 2008: 171). In some cases in which insurers opted to cover the drug, it was not at preferred rates, meaning that patients were saddled with higher copayments. As Dr. Andrew L. Smith, medical director of heart failure and transplantation at Emory Healthcare in Atlanta, put it, "BiDil has been farther down the [formulary] chain with most insurance carriers, so coverage for the medicine without a substantial co-pay has been a problem and the medication is expensive" (Kreimer 2007). Some BiDil advocates have suggested that the failure of insurers to cover BiDil has less to do with costs and more to do with the health care system's generally poor treatment of African Americans. In a scathing letter, Juan Cofield, president of the NAACP's New England council, chided the Boston regional office of the Centers for Medicare and Medicaid Services (CMS) for failing to promote insurance coverage of BiDil. He stated that Medicare's stance "is so contrary to evidence-based medicine and so extraordinary that it arouses suspicions of institutional racism" (Winstein 2007). In an interview with the *Wall Street Journal*, Cofield added that if BiDil "were not a medication for blacks, [CMS's] response would be different" (Winstein 2007). Whatever the motive for insurers passing over covering BiDil, the burden of high out-of-pocket expenses is believed to have made the drug prohibitively expensive for many patients.

Another reason, no doubt, for BiDil's market failure is patient mistrust and the unpalatability of a drug just for blacks (Roberts 2011b, Pollock 2012, Kahn 2013). Although BiDil received substantial support from African American organizations and leaders, there were sectors of the black population, including patients, who were highly suspicious of the drug. A cartoon in Keith Knight's weekly syndicated comic strip *The K Chronicles* poignantly illustrates this mistrust (Knight 2005). The first panel shows four black individuals looking suspiciously at a bottle of BiDil that is sitting in the middle of a table. One says, "I ain't gonna try it. ... You try it!!" Another responds, "No way!! I ain't gonna try it!!" A caption on the right side reads, "BiDil, the first government approved drug specifically made for a particular race, is supposed to help black folks combat heart failure." The next panel reminds readers about the history of US experimentation on black bodies. There are references to the Tuskegee syphilis experiment, eugenic sterilization, and radiation experiments.[10] The caption states, "Now ... given the United States government's less than stellar track record concerning the health of its black citizens ... It's really no surprise that folks may be a bit reluctant to try the drug." A final panel suggests that BiDil will be remembered as a gross error: "I can't wait to hear the apology the Senate will give 50 years from now for the infamous BiDil 'mistake.'"

This mistrust toward race-specific drugs is not simply a matter of popular culture. A study by Celeste Condit and colleagues (2003) on patient attitudes concerning pharmacogenetic medicine determined that such mistrust was quite prevalent in the black community.[11] The study oversampled for African Americans and found that respondents "would be highly suspicious of race-labeled drugs; with 47.5% saying they would be very suspicious of their safety and 40.6% indicating they would be very suspicious of their efficacy" (Condit et al. 2003: 385). This suspicion is connected not only to past medical experimentation on blacks but also to the history of segregated and unequal medical treatment. When it comes to medical care, "black only" has traditionally meant inferior or potentially dangerous (Roberts 2011b). Given black suspicion about race-based drugs, then, it is not surprising that BiDil failed to reach its market. Indeed, for many blacks the drug was apparently not palatable.

In addition to price and mistrust, physician skepticism also appears to have played a role in BiDil's demise (Kahn 2013). A study by Danielle Frank and colleagues (2010) of 90 general internists found that these physicians were generally wary of race-based therapies and of BiDil in particular.[12] Physician skepticism revolved principally around the underlying premise of race-based drugs. The authors note:

> Many physicians voiced concern that prescribing medications based on race presumes that some inherent patient factor influencing drug responses differs in meaningful ways by racial group. They were wary that the category of race would be able to capture differences at the genetic level.

---

10 On the Tuskegee syphilis experiment, see Reverby 2009, on the eugenic sterilization of African American men and women, see Roberts 1997, and on the radiation experiments on black bodies, see Washington 2006.

11 Other studies have confirmed that distrust of race-based pharmaceuticals is widespread among African Americans. See De Marco 2010 and Butrick et al. 2011.

12 Physician attitudes toward race-based therapies were not totally negative. Some expressed the belief that certain medications, ACE inhibitors in particular, did work differently depending on race.

> The physicians' skepticism of race-based therapies was based, in part, on their belief that the link between race and genetics is inexact because racial intermixing has resulted in a sharing of clinically meaningful genotypes. Instead of using race as a placeholder for genetic variation, physicians advocated examining the genetic polymorphism that may account for differential responses to drug therapy. [Frank et al. 2010: 385, 388]

Physicians were also concerned about the medical and social implications of race-based therapeutics. Some worried that attributing health disparities to genetic differences between racial groups could be used as an excuse to dismiss social and environmental factors in disease causality. As one physician put it,

> What I don't want to happen is that race is used as an excuse for why there are differences or disparities. Well, there [are] more blacks in renal failure because they have uncontrolled hypertension because they are made up that way which allows us to dismiss all the environmental issues. That is my fear with the way we are moving toward development of race-specific drugs. [Frank et al. 2010: 387]

With respect to BiDil, physicians evinced even stronger skepticism. As Frank and her colleagues (2010: 388) state, "Black and white physicians cited market forces as the primary impetus behind its creation. Physicians overwhelmingly voiced concern that commercial considerations shaped the development of the first drug approved for a race-specific indication. Most physicians did not feel that BiDil represented the future direction of race-based therapies." Such a high level of physician skepticism toward BiDil, and toward race-based therapies in general, could most certainly have contributed to the low prescription rates of the drug.

Finally, NitroMed's marketing strategy also likely contributed to BiDil's failure (Pollock 2012, Kahn 2013). A key part of the company's approach, as I have discussed, involved targeting black consumers. The hope was that patients would absorb the publicity about BiDil and prevail on physicians to prescribe the drug to them. The problem with this approach is that it presumes an ideal subject position that African Americans cannot easily embody—that of the active patient-consumer. Active patient-consumers are individuals who take upon themselves the primary responsibility for managing their health. They actively and responsibly search for health information and use the knowledge they gain to negotiate therapy and produce health (Barbot 2006, Briggs and Hallin 2007). The issue is that physicians do not necessarily imagine or treat African Americans as active patient-consumers. Instead, blacks are often cast as problem patients. For example, a study by Rose Clark-Hitt and colleagues (2010) found that physicians and nurses generally explained racial disparities in health treatment in terms of African American patients' perceived shortcomings, including "Black patients' lack of compliance with treatment, not being as informed as White patients, taking less control over their own care, distrust, missing appointments, substance abuse, and hesitance to accept referrals to specialists" (Clark-Hitt et al. 2010: 390). Given that health care providers tend to see them as difficult patients, African Americans are not well positioned to make consumerist demands on doctors. Indeed, insofar as blacks are not seen as embodying the ideal of the active patient-consumer, physicians are not likely to listen to them when they make demands (Pollock 2012). A marketing strategy that relies on reaching physicians through targeting black patients thus faces an uphill battle to succeed. In the case of NitroMed, it appears that the hill was too high to climb.

Continuing Value of Race

Although BiDil did not do well in the marketplace, this failure does not appear to have hampered the use of race in biomedical research and pharmaceutical development. In fact, the interest in race-based therapies appears to have accelerated (Roberts 2011b, Kahn 2013). We can see the continuing value of race in at least three domains: patent protection, drug product differentiation, and racial dosing. With respect to patents, Jonathan Kahn (2013) conducted an analysis of gene-related patents issued and patent applications filed between 1976 and 2007. He determined that there has been a significant trend toward using racial and ethnic categories in such patents, the trend being the result of both the large amounts of genetic information that have been produced in the wake of the Human Genome Project and the federal requirement to use racial and ethnic categories in drug development and clinical trials. Kahn specifically found that the number of race-inflected patents issued went from 0 between 1976 and 1997 to 29 between 1998 and 2007 (Kahn 2013: 131). As for patent applications filed, the number that included race-related terms was 151 between 2001 and 2007, with 86 being filed between 2006 and 2007 alone (Kahn 2013: 132). The terms used in these patents include *race*, *ethnic*, *African American/black*, *Asian*, *Caucasian/white*, *Hispanic/Latino*, *Native American*, and *Pacific Islander*.

The proliferation of racial patents and patent applications is highly significant. It signals that biotechnology and pharmaceutical companies are following in NitroMed's footsteps and seeking to develop products targeted to particular races (Roberts 2011b). There are numerous cases that can be used to exemplify this trend. Here I highlight three examples. One application filed in 2012 seeks to patent a method "of diagnosing susceptibility to insulin resistance in *Hispanic* Americans by determining the presence of a risk haplotype at the LPL locus, the LPIN1 locus, and/or elevated levels of gamma-glutamyl transferase" (Rotter et al. 2012). The patent is partly based on a study conducted by the inventors that purports to show that the LPL gene, which encodes for lipoprotein lipase, is a common genetic determinant for liver enzymes and insulin resistance in US Hispanic populations. Another application, this one filed in 2010, seeks to patent a combination therapy consisting of telaprevir and pegylated interferon alfa-2a to treat Latino and African American patients infected with the hepatitis C virus (McNair 2010). It rests on research showing "that telaprevir-based regimens lead to improved viral responses in African Americans and Latinos as compared to [standard] therapy alone" (McNair 2010). A third application, also filed in 2010, seeks to patent "methods of prophylaxis therapy for MI [myocardial infarction] in human subjects having a race including black *African* ancestry by administering to the subject a composition comprising a therapeutically effective amount of MI therapeutic agent that inhibits leukotriene synthesis in vivo" (Helgadottir et al. 2010). The application is based on research indicating that "African Americans are an especially promising target population for ... anti-leukotriene therapies" (Helgadottir et al. 2010). Uniting these three patents is the assumption that there is something fundamentally different, and potentially genetically-based, about racial groups that warrants targeting products just to them. Moreover, they all invoke race as a way to gain market protection and potentially generate vital value (Roberts 2011b).

Besides being used in patents, race is also being employed as a way to differentiate pharmaceutical products in a crowed marketplace (Roberts 2011b, Kahn 2013). The idea here is simply that pharmaceutical companies are racially branding their medicines as a way of differentiating them from similar products. A key example is the drug Travatan. Manufactured by the eye care company Alcon, this drug was approved by the FDA in 2001 for treating intraocular pressure due to glaucoma or other eye diseases. Clinical trials suggested that Travatan was highly effective at reducing pressure inside the eye in all patients: subjects treated with the drug experienced 7 to 8 mm Hg reductions in intraocular pressure (Alcon 2013). When broken into subgroups, the data showed that the drug worked especially well on African Americans: the mean intraocular pressure reduction in black patients was up to 1.8 mm Hg greater than in nonblacks. Travatan's package insert notes that it is not clear whether the difference in the drug's effectiveness "is due to race or to heavily pigmented irides" (Alcon 2013). Nevertheless, Alcon has conspicuously employed race in its marketing of the drug, developing campaigns specifically for African Americans. For example, through Travatan® Project Focus, the company gave free glaucoma screenings at local churches, community centers, and major cultural events to at-risk African American patients (Alcon 2003). At these forums, Alcon also distributed materials on glaucoma and Travatan to educate blacks about eye health. In its targeting of African Americans, Alcon's pitch involved touting the benefits of Travatan for this population. In a press release about Travatan® Project Focus, the company noted:

> Glaucoma is the leading cause of blindness among African-Americans. It affects them at a younger age and frequently results in rapid and severe vision loss. Elevated intraocular pressure is a risk factor associated with glaucoma. Travatan® ophthalmic solution is a glaucoma medication from Alcon that has proven to be more effective in lowering intraocular pressure in African-Americans than in non-African-Americans. [Alcon 2003]

Alcon, then, sought to differentiate Travatan from other glaucoma drugs by claiming it worked particularly well on a specific race: African Americans.

Another important example of a racially marked product is the beta blocker Bystolic, the brand name for the generic nebivolol (Kahn 2009, 2013). Marketed by Forest Laboratories, the drug is approved for the treatment of hypertension. The market for beta blockers in the United States is highly competitive, with at least 18 beta blockers available to consumers (Kahn 2013). Like Alcon, Forest Laboratories has turned to race to differentiate its drug from the competition. Specifically, the company has emphasized that Bystolic works well in African Americans (Forest Laboratories 2007). This claim is based on results from a clinical trial that examined Bystolic in self-identified African Americans (Saunders et al. 2007). A press release from Forest Laboratories succinctly describes the trial and its results:

> In this 12-week double-blind trial, 300 African-American patients with stage I-II hypertension were randomly assigned to receive once-daily placebo or nebivolol at a 2.5, 5, 10, 20, or 40 mg dose. Among the 259 patients who completed the 12-week therapy, by comparison to placebo treatment, nebivolol significantly reduced sitting diastolic blood pressure at all daily doses greater than or equal to 5 mg and sitting systolic blood pressure at all daily doses greater than or equal to 10 mg with a low rate of side effects. [2007]

The claim that Bystolic works well in African Americans is significant because there has been strong indication in the medical literature that beta blockers are not particularly effective in treating high blood pressure in this population (Veiga and Taylor 1986, Gibbs, Beevers, and Lip 1999). This point was emphasized by the lead investigator of the Bystolic clinical trial, Elijah Saunders: "Advances like this in the beta blocker class are particularly important because African Americans have an historically poor response to beta blocker therapy for hypertension" (Forest Laboratories 2007). On the basis of this claim of efficacy in African Americans, Forest Laboratories was thus able to set Bystolic apart from other beta blockers. The company even succeeded in having its racial efficacy claim included in the FDA-approved prescription label for the drug. The label reads, "Effectiveness was established in Blacks" (Forest Laboratories 2011).

A final domain in which race continues to be significant is racial dosing. The idea here is that different racial groups need to be prescribed different doses of certain drugs because they react to drugs differently. The drugs warfarin and rosuvastatin are important examples (Roberts 2011b, Kahn 2013). Warfarin, marketed by Bristol-Myers Squibb under the name Coumadin, is a blood-thinning drug widely prescribed for preventing blood clots. Medical researchers have observed that there is some variation in how different racial groups respond to the drug (Johnson 2008). Compared to whites, for example, Asians on average metabolize warfarin at faster rates. This means that Asians typically require smaller doses than whites to achieve similar effects. Given such observations, the FDA approved a prescription label for Coumadin that contains a section on Asian patients that reads, "Asian patients may require lower initiation and maintenance doses of warfarin" (Bristol-Myers Squibb 2011). Similarly, the cholesterol-lowering drug rosuvastatin, marketed by AstraZeneca as Crestor, is believed to have different effects on Asians compared to other populations. As with Coumadin, the FDA approved a racially inflected label for this drug. For example, in a section on clinical pharmacology, the label notes,

> A population pharmacokinetic analysis revealed no clinically relevant differences in pharmacokinetics among Caucasian, Hispanic, and Black or Afro-Caribbean groups. However, pharmacokinetic studies, including one conducted in the US, have demonstrated an approximate 2-fold elevation in median exposure (AUC and C_{max}) in Asian subjects when compared with a Caucasian control group. [AstraZeneca 2013]

The label also includes a separate section that addresses dosage in Asian patients, recommending that doctors start them with a daily dose of 5 mg as opposed to the standard 10 to 20 mg.

For both warfarin and rosuvastatin, it is extremely important that patients receive the right doses. For example, patients receiving too much warfarin are at risk of hemorrhaging, while those receiving too little of the drug face the possibility of blood clots and stroke. In the case of rosuvastatin, high doses of the drug have been known to cause rhabdomyolysis, a rare condition in which muscle cells break down. Highlighting the importance of correct dosing is the fact that warfarin is the medication most commonly implicated in emergency hospitalizations for adverse drug events in US adults 65 years of age or older (Budnitz et al. 2011). From 2007 through 2009, warfarin accounted for 33 percent of such hospitalizations. Given this context, racial dosing would appear to be an appropriate practice aimed at mitigating adverse drug reactions. However, as Dorothy Roberts asks with respect to rosuvastatin, "if the usual starting dosage of Crestor can be toxic for some patients, is race the most accurate way to determine the right amount?" (2011b: 193). Her answer is a resounding no. She argues that it is not good medical practice to base dosing decisions on a social category. If there is a genotype that increases the levels of Crestor in the body, it is not race specific. Other populations—Latinos, whites, blacks, and so forth—would also have the genotype and would potentially suffer injury from ingesting the standard recommended dose. Such patients should really be given the lower starting dose recommended for Asian patients. The way to determine the right dosing need for patients is not to resort to race but to develop tests that can identify whether an individual, regardless of race, carries the risky genotype. In the absence of such a test, all patients should be started at safe lower doses. Of course, if doctors were to prescribe Crestor at lower amounts, this would undoubtedly hurt AstraZeneca's profits. Race is thus valuable here as a way to reduce doses for some patients while keeping them high for most.

Conclusion

As this chapter has made clear, the fostering of bodily vitality and the economization of life are closely intertwined. Indeed, the production of health is very much connected to the generation of wealth. In such a milieu, the life of the racial body has become a key potential source of economic value, that is, of racial vital value. BiDil is an important case in point. There is no doubt that the purpose of the drug has been to nurture the vitality of the African American body. On the basis of the available evidence, the drug clearly saves lives. However, BiDil has also been used to generate profits. Commercial factors were unquestionably a motivating force behind the transformation of the drug into a racial pharmaceutical. The production of BiDil has thus been not just about saving black lives but also about salvaging the drug itself in order to generate profits. Ultimately, the drug has not delivered on its economic promise. Its high price, mistrust on the part of patients, physician skepticism, and NitroMed's flawed marketing strategy have all combined to make BiDil a commercial failure. Its lack of success, however, has not dampened the drive to use race in medicine. Pharmaceutical and biotechnology companies continue to believe that there are profits to be made from cultivating the life of racial bodies. It is likely only a matter of time before we see another racialized drug on the horizon.

Chapter 6
Neoliberalization of Life

The argument I have advanced in this book is that racialized pharmaceuticals need to be located within the biopolitics of the twenty-first century. This is a politics whose aim clearly is to foster life. Concentrating on BiDil, I have suggested that racialized drugs are undeniably about cultivating the life of the racial body. Indeed, BiDil's advocates—from NitroMed and the NAACP to the Association for Black Cardiologists—have all seen the drug as life-saving technology. On some level, then, BiDil is fundamentally linked to questions of rights and citizenship. The racialization of this drug is about the right of a socially marginalized population, namely African Americans, to have access to the advantages of biomedicine. I have also noted, however, that although BiDil might bring the benefits of modern medicine to African Americans and thereby help to prolong black lives, the drug's vital politics also has a potentially exclusionary underside. A central problem is the way in which African Americans have been geneticized as a result of BiDil. Basically, the FDA's approval of the drug only for blacks gives the mistaken impression that this population somehow constitutes a distinct genetic grouping. Also problematic is NitroMed's effort to capitalize on racial life. Although pharmaceutical products clearly aim to foster the vitality of the body, they also seek to produce economic value. In the case of BiDil, the drug was in some ways less about saving black lives and more about the profits to be derived from tapping racial markets. The upshot, then, is that although BiDil's vital politics are on the side of life, the drug nevertheless has troublesome elements.

In this final chapter, I situate BiDil and racialized medicine in the context of what might be called the *neoliberalization of life* (see also Waldby and Cooper 2008). Since the 1970s, there has been a general reconfiguration of the territory of government in the United States (Rose 1999, Inda 2006). Put briefly, the model of the welfare state, which was dominant in some guise for much of the twentieth century, has generally given way to that of the neoliberal state. Under this new model, political government generally no longer acts to safeguard the life and well-being of the population by maintaining a realm of collective security. Social insurance programs, defined as those public mechanisms through which the state sought to insure individuals against life's insecurities, have thus largely vanished and been replaced by a system of marketized and individualized risk management. Indeed, by means of the market, individuals are now expected to take upon themselves the principal responsibility for managing their own security and that of their loved ones. They are counted on to assume an entrepreneurial outlook toward life and to independently insure themselves against the problems of ill health, accidental loss, unemployment, and anything else that could potentially threaten their well-being. In a neoliberal context, then, the fostering of life takes place not through a benevolent state but via individual initiative. Indeed, the neoliberal state exercises only limited powers of its own when it comes to the social protection of the population. A major consequence of the neoliberalization of life—of shifting the responsibility for nurturing the welfare of the population from the state to individuals—has been to render life precarious, as people are left to fend for themselves against the insecurities of living.[1] In this chapter, I explore how BiDil and racialized medicine partake in this neoliberal context.

From Welfarism to Neoliberalism

For much of the twentieth century, political government in the United States was underpinned by a distinct political mentality that has come to be called *welfarism* (Dean 1999, Rose 1999). Welfarism was grounded in the belief that the state should maintain a realm of collective security in order to safeguard the life of each and every member of the population. It was based on the idea that the situation of all social groups within society—workers, employers, professionals, and managers—could simultaneously and gradually be improved. Programmatically, welfarism targeted a range of distinct problem domains: the living and working conditions of the laboring classes; the sexuality, health, and education of children; the norms of family life; the role of women as mothers and housewives; poverty and squalor; prostitution and immorality; delinquency and antisocial behavior; and so forth. The government's goal in administering these domains was to ensure collective vitality by curtailing the risks to individuals and families that resulted from the viccissitudes of economic cycles, alleviating the harmful consequences of unrestrained economic activity by interceding directly in the conditions of employment, and generally promoting the betterment of the social and biological lives of individuals (Castel 1999, Rose 2000a).

The principle means by which the welfarist—or, simply, welfare—state sought to ensure collective vitality was social insurance, which took many forms, from accident insurance and unemployment benefits to health and safety legislation. The goal was essentially to secure the life of the population against the risks associated with such phenomena as poverty, old age, sickness, unemployment, accidents, crime, and ill health. Social insurance was thus an

1 On the precarity of life in general, see Judith Butler 2004.

inclusive and solidaristic governmental practice. As Nikolas Rose notes, "it incarnate[d] social solidarity in collectivizing the management of the individual and collective dangers posed by the economic riskiness of a capricious system of wage labor, and the corporeal riskiness of a body subject to sickness and injury, under the stewardship of a [welfare] State" (1996b: 48). Put otherwise, social insurance was deployed as a mechanism of solidarity that translated accidents, sickness, unemployment, and other afflictions into insurable risks that were individually remunerated but collectively borne. It provided a certain measure of individual and collective security against the uncertainties of social life. Notably, this allocation of social provisions to individuals on the basis of their membership in a collectivity embodied a particular conception of the subject of government. The political subject was conceptualized as a social citizen, a being whose life and health were guaranteed through collective dependencies and solidarities. Indeed, the individual was ordained into society in the figure of a citizen with social rights and needs (Miller and Rose 1990). Welfarism, then, conceived of the subject as an individual who was to be "governed through society," within a nexus of collective responsibility (Rose 1996b: 40). It constructed citizenship in terms of contentment, solidarity, and the obligation of the state to foster individual and collective life.

In the mid-1970s, welfarism came under severe attack from a variety of political forces (Rose 2000a). Neoliberals asserted the necessity of moving away from the excessive governing that is characteristic of the welfare state to a more frugal form of governance—one that would foster the mechanisms of the market and thus allow economic processes to operate naturally; civil libertarians expressed concern about the incompatibility between the discretionary powers of social government and the rights of individuals; and those on the left questioned the social state's effectiveness in minimizing ill health, poverty, and insecurity. Whatever their other incongruities, all sides seemed to agree that the role of the state as guarantor of steadfast and progressive social advancement had become deeply problematic. The welfare state—with its large bureaucracies, extravagant welfare programs, and interventionist social engineering—had simply become excessive. It not only hindered the market, created costly and inept bureaucracies, and generated exorbitant taxes, but worse, instead of fostering social responsibility and citizenship, it actually created dependency and a client mentality, thus heightening the very problems of delinquency, immorality, and ill health that it meant to remedy.

A major outcome of the critique of welfarism has been the gradual reshaping of the terrain of government in the United States (O'Malley 1992, Dean 1999, Rose 1999). Today, welfarism is no longer the principle mentality underpinning political government. It has generally been replaced by neoliberalism. Under this new mentality, political government no longer appears obligated to tackle all the ills of social and economic life by fostering a sphere of collective security.

The responsibility for dealing with the problems of living has largely been displaced from the state to a multitude of specific actors: individuals, schools, communities, localities, hospitals, charities, and so forth. Social insurance, as a socializing and collectivizing principle of solidarity, has thus generally given way to the privatized administration of risk. Market instruments—contracts, consumers, and competition—play a crucial role here. It is through the market that individual actors are expected to foster their own lives and secure their own well-being. Indeed, the market has become the preferred mechanism for safeguarding the life of the population—for averting the risks linked to old age, ill health, sickness, poverty, and accidents. For example, there has been a proliferation of market-based, semi-autonomous nonstate organizations whose role is to administer areas of social life formerly under the direct sway of the state. The functions for which such organizations have taken responsibility include planning the regeneration and government of urban locales; managing formerly public utilities such as water, gas, and electricity; regulating investment and securities in the financial sector; and providing welfare, prison, and police services (Rose 1996b: 56). Neoliberalism, then, entails new modes of apportioning the work of government among the political apparatus, communities, economic actors, and private citizens. It seeks to govern not through society but, as Nikolas Rose argues, "through the regulated choices of individual citizens, now construed as subjects of choices and aspirations to self-actualization and self-fulfillment" (1996b: 41). Here the state, instead of being a provider—the ultimate guarantor of security—exercises limited authority with respect to fostering individual and collective vitality, and thus the public provision of social protection ceases to appear necessary to governing well.

Like welfarism, neoliberalism depends on a certain conception of the persons to be subjected to government. The political subject under neoliberalism is not a social citizen whose security is guaranteed through the bonds of collective solidarity and the receipt of public largesse, but rather an autonomous individual whose citizenship is derived from active self-promotion and self-actualization (O'Malley 1999, Rose 1999, 2000a, Brown 2003, Wacquant 2010). Indeed, the neoliberal citizen is expected to be an entrepreneur unto him- or herself: each individual is to maximize the quality of his or her own life—and give meaning and value to it—through acts of responsible choice. Citizens are thus now exhorted to take upon themselves the primary responsibility for fostering their own lives and those of their loved ones. They are asked to adopt a calculative and prudent disposition toward risk and not to rely on socialized securities. For example, neoliberal citizens are supposed to provide for their own retirement through private pension plans; secure themselves against ill health, unemployment, and accidental loss through private insurance; and generally play a big part in safeguarding themselves from anything that could potentially endanger the safety of their freely chosen way of life (Rose 1999). Neoliberalism, then, rests on the reconstitution of the political subject from a social being with rights and needs to a neoliberal citizen with choices and yearnings toward self-fulfillment. It is a mentality of governance that works to responsibilize individuals for their own care and well-being. As such, neoliberalism is essentially about making ethical subjects. The term *ethical* here refers not so much to moral practices as to how persons conduct themselves and comprehend their existence. It speaks to the duty of individuals to take proper care of themselves. In a neoliberal context, ethical beings are ones who assume charge of their own lives and adopt a prudent disposition toward the future. They are persons who comport themselves rationally and responsibly.

To sum up, neoliberalism envisions securing the life of the population not through strategies directed and financed by the state, but through the instrumentalization of a desire for self-reliance—through the production of prudent, self-managing, ethical political subjects. It is a political mentality that constitutes citizens, as Pat O'Malley notes, not "as members of an overarching social whole, to which they owe allegiance, and to which they can make a legitimate call for social assistance," but "as autonomous individuals, responsible for their own fate, invested with personal agency and thus with a purely personal responsibility for their status and actions" (1999: 95). The characteristic elements of the neoliberal reconfiguration of government in the United States thus include the downscaling of the state (with respect to social protection), the privatization of numerous services formerly part of the state apparatus, the devolution of power to communities and localities, and the constitution of the political subject as a responsible and entrepreneurial individual (Rose 1996c, Osborne and Rose 1999, Brown 2003, Wacquant 2010). In short, neoliberalism seeks to place a limit on what the state can do for individuals. It endeavors to govern by making citizens individually responsible for securing their own life, health, and happiness.

The Precarization of Life

The shift from welfarism to neoliberalism has had far-reaching effects on the health and welfare of the population in the United States. David Harvey has noted that, "[a]s the state withdraws from welfare provision and diminishes its role in arenas such as health care, public education, and social services, which were once so fundamental to embedded liberalism, it leaves larger and larger segments of the population exposed to impoverishment" (2005: 76). A major consequence of neoliberalism has thus been the precarization of life. The basic problem with this political mentality is that it depoliticizes social problems. As Wendy Brown has argued, "[a]s neoliberalism converts every political and social problem into market terms, it converts them to individual problems with market solutions" (2006: 704). Examples include the introduction of charter schools, private schools, and voucher systems as a way to deal with the crumbling quality of public education; boutique medicine as a reaction to the erosion of health care provision; and private security guards and gated communities as a response to the social insecurity produced by rising economic inequality. So, rather than providing collective solutions to socially and politically produced problems—whether to improve public education, strengthen the health care system for everyone, or offset the destructive effects of economic cycles in order to ensure collective welfare and reduce social inequality—neoliberalism leaves it to individuals to fend for themselves using the mechanisms of the market. However, individuals are quite often not in a position to deal with social problems all by themselves; as a result their lives are rendered more insecure and vulnerable.

To illustrate how neoliberalism has made life more precarious, we can examine the fate of War on Poverty and Great Society welfare programs such as Aid to Families with Dependent Children (AFDC). During the last few decades of the twentieth century, welfare programs came under attack from all sides of the political spectrum for having worsened, instead of ameliorated, the problem of poverty. "We tried to provide more for the poor," asserted conservative academic Charles A. Murray, "and produced more poor instead. We tried to remove the barriers to escape from poverty, and inadvertently built a trap" (1984: 9). The basic issue with welfare programs, according to critics, was that they had induced the poor into a state of dependency. For many detractors, dependency was indeed at the heart of welfare's problems. Democratic Senator Daniel Patrick Moynihan, for example, noted that

> the issue of welfare is the issue of dependency. It is different from poverty. To be poor is an objective condition; to be dependent, a subjective one as well. ... Being poor is often associated with considerable personal qualities; being dependent rarely so. [Dependency] is an incomplete state in life: normal in the child, abnormal in the adult. In a world where completed men and women stand on their own feet, persons who are dependent—as the buried imagery of the word denotes—hang. [Moynihan 1973: 17]

The term *dependency* here has two important registers, one economic, the other ethical. From an economic standpoint, *dependency* simply points to how the poor—impoverished unwed mothers in particular—had come to rely on the state, instead of work, as their primary source of subsistence. The contention was that welfare programs, AFDC in particular, had made it possible and acceptable for the poor to "choose" the road of unemployment. The poor were thus imagined as rational economic actors who had calculated that they could use the welfare system for their own benefit and earn a living without having to work (Rose 2000b). From an ethical standpoint, *dependency* refers to how relying on the state for one's subsistence turned out to be a habit-forming practice that in the long run stripped the poor of their self-discipline and of their competence to function as responsible adults. It points to how the receipt of welfare inculcated the poor with a client mentality and turned them into passive, lazy individuals who had no capacity for work or ethical self-management. Far from helping the poor, then, what welfare programs did, according to critics, was create a class of economically and ethically suspect citizens who were locked into poverty. They produced an underclass of dependent subjects bereft of moral character, lacking dignity and autonomy, and unwilling or unable to be self-sufficient and to take individual responsibility for their own care. The archetype of this new class was the welfare mother (also known more derogatorily as the welfare queen), imagined as a licentious young, black, single, inner-city woman prone to bearing babies she could not support (Fraser 1993).

Given the general consensus that welfare programs had failed the poor, especially black single mothers, political authorities devised numerous schemes to reform the welfare system. These schemes generally took the ethical reconstitution of welfare subjects as their primary task. They sought to reactivate the autonomous capabilities of such citizens in order to get them off welfare and reinsert them into circuits of responsible self-management. The most significant reform scheme was undoubtedly the Personal Responsibility and Work Opportunity Reconciliation Act of 1996 (the Welfare Act). The ambitious objective of the Welfare Act was essentially to eliminate welfare dependency or, as former President Bill Clinton so famously put it, to "end welfare as we know it" (1993). It sought to accomplish this aim primarily through making the reformation of conduct a condition for receiving benefits (Abramovitz 2000, Schram 2000). Pragmatically, this effort entailed dismantling AFDC and replacing it with Temporary Assistance for Needy Families (TANF). AFDC was an entitlement program that guaranteed cash assistance to poor, female-headed families whose income and assets fell below a preestablished threshold. There were generally no other stipulations—such as work participation or time limits—attached to the receipt of such aid. Families could obtain assistance in perpetuity, as long as they met the income eligibility requirements. TANF, on the other hand, is not an entitlement program. This means that poor families are no longer automatically entitled to receive cash assistance if their income falls beneath a certain level. They now have to satisfy several additional conditions. Two are particularly important to highlight here. The first has to do with behavior: TANF makes the receipt of aid conditional upon work. Poor families can obtain assistance without any reciprocal obligations for two years. After that, the parent must be engaged in work or work-related activities (for example, schooling, vocational training, and skill development) in order to continue receiving benefits. The other condition has to do with time: TANF imposes temporal limits on the receipt of aid. Citizens can be on welfare for no more than five years of their life. Behind the imposition of these new conditions is the idea that the most effective way to end welfare dependency is to require recipients to find a job as rapidly as possible and to develop an aptitude for work through hands-on training. Work is key because it is assumed to confer independence, in both economic and ethical terms. With respect to the former, work is seen as allowing welfare subjects to become financially autonomous; in regard to the latter, work is believed to capacitate welfare recipients with the self-esteem they need in order to more generally take charge of their lives. The goal here is thus to nurture and restore self-sufficiency and autonomy, to handle welfare subjects in a way that prepares them to assume responsibility for their own well-being, and to turn them into productive members of society.

Crucial to TANF's responsibilizing strategy is the careful monitoring of welfare subjects (Schram 2000), principally through intensive case management. Such micro-administration entails at least two important activities. The first, and perhaps most important, of these is the screening of welfare applicants. The main purpose of screening is to ascertain the job readiness of individuals seeking benefits. The focus here is not so much on assessing their specific job skills and training needs as on determining their behavioral and psychological capacity to function in the workplace, because it is personal deficiencies—habits, behaviors, and personal characteristics—and not lack of job skills that are considered to be the primary impediment to being job-ready. Significant screening practices accordingly include checking for alcohol abuse, mental disorders, drug use, and other conditions presumed to hamper an individual's ability to self-govern. Should claimants be deemed incapable of self-sufficiency, the charge of welfare management is to determine what kinds of collateral services—counseling, psychological, and so forth—they need in order to deal with their personal shortcomings and thus become ready for the world of work. Should welfare seekers be judged competent, however, the job of the welfare administration shifts to pushing them immediately into the labor market and deflecting them from getting benefits.

The second case management activity entails making welfare recipients sign individual responsibility plans. Known in some states as contracts of mutual responsibility, these plans essentially amount to social contracts whereby society agrees to aid the individual in her time of need on the condition that she promises to take measures that will lead her toward a paying job. The fact that these plans are contracts is not accidental. The idea here is that requiring welfare recipients to enter into a binding agreement will likely make them more accountable for carrying through with programs for achieving self-sufficiency.

Significantly, supporters of welfare reform have touted TANF as a great success (Seccombe and Hoffman 2007). They have argued that the program has empowered welfare subjects to reconstitute themselves ethically: to enter the labor market, successfully take up the care of themselves and their loved ones, and leave behind a life of dependency. "[W]elfare reform," notes Tommy G. Thompson, former Secretary of the Department of Health and Human Services, "is moving more people into work so that they can support themselves and their families. . . . [It] has helped an unprecedented number of people on welfare to become self-supporting" (Jackson 2001: A14). The Heritage Foundation, a conservative think tank, has made similar claims: "The 1996 welfare reform legislation made remarkable headway in helping welfare dependents to move toward self-sufficiency. It dramatically reduced the caseload of dependents, reduced child poverty, and increased employment among single mothers" (Rector 2004). The main evidence that welfare reform advocates highlight as signaling the empowerment of welfare subjects is the ever-diminishing welfare rolls. In California, for instance, the number of individual welfare recipients dropped from about 2.58 million in August 1996 to a little more than 1.27 million in June 2000 (US DHHS 2000b). Nationwide, the numbers dropped from 12.24 to 5.78 million over the same period (US DHHS 2000b). Today, the numbers are even lower. In June 2013 about 3.68 million people nationwide received TANF benefits (US DHHS 2013).

This triumphant take on welfare reform is correct in one respect: there has certainly been a sharp decline in welfare caseloads. However, it is not necessarily the case that those people who have "left" welfare have become empowered and triumphantly self-supporting (Abramovitz 2000, Mink 1998, Schram 2000). For example, women are routinely expelled from the welfare rolls for failing to meet the goals set out in their individual responsibility plans (King 1999). Their specific infractions range from simple offenses such as skipping appointments with caseworkers to more serious transgressions such as failing to take steps to find, procure, and hold a job (Schram 2000). From the perspective of welfare reformers, the punishment such women receive is well deserved: they have essentially failed to show that they can become responsible individuals. From the viewpoint of welfare advocates, though, the castigation is overly severe, for it is not necessarily the case that such women are deliberately "irresponsible." There are actually numerous objective barriers that can block their path to self-sufficiency. For instance, employers are often reluctant to hire them (Berrick 2001: 138). One reason for this reluctance is the general stereotyping of welfare women as lazy and unreliable; another reason is that such women unfortunately often lack the vocational skills necessary to make them attractive to employers. Other barriers include such factors as lack of jobs in the inner city, the absence of good public transportation to shuttle women to areas where jobs are more readily available, insufficient access to the training and schooling needed for social advancement, and the dearth of affordable child care (Schneiderman and Schneiderman 2001: M2). Whether the punishment is just or harsh, the fact remains that many women have been summarily dismissed from receiving welfare. Their fate: to join the ranks of the homeless, to survive on informal businesses—such as providing in-home child care and braiding hair—that previously supplemented their welfare income, and to exist on the charity of family members, churches, community organizations, and so forth (King 1999, Rose 1999, Abramovitz 2000).

It is also important to note that even those people who have left welfare for gainful employment have not necessarily become gloriously self-sufficient. In fact, such individuals generally end up in low-wage jobs that offer few, if any, benefits (Acs and Loprest 2004a, Seccombe and Hoffman 2007). In their review of state and regional studies dealing with the employment and well-being of former welfare families, Acs and Loprest (2004b) calculated that the mean hourly wage paid to welfare leavers ranged from $7.50 to $8.74. These are basically poverty wages. Notably, not only do the occupations of welfare leavers tend to pay poorly, but their employers generally do not offer health insurance. A study drawing on data from the Urban Institute's National Survey of America's Families found that in both 1999 and 2002 only about a third of working welfare leavers had employer-sponsored health insurance (Loprest 2003). Given their low wages and lack of health benefits (which are provided under TANF), many former welfare recipients are left struggling to survive (Seccombe and Hoffman 2007). Indeed, as Acs and Loprest (2004b) point out in their review, at least a third of former TANF recipients experienced food scarcity after leaving the program, with about a fifth receiving emergency food aid. They further note that between 25 and 50 percent of ex-TANF families struggled to pay their rent and utility bills, with some having their utilities shut off due to failure to pay. Being self-sufficient is thus not as empowering as advocates of welfare reform suggest.

The reality of welfare reform is that it has not necessarily improved the lives of former welfare subjects. In fact, for many, life has become more insecure. A study by the National Poverty Center reports that the number of US households living in extreme poverty—defined as surviving on $2 or less per person per day—more than doubled between 1996 and 2011, increasing from 636,000 to 1.46 million (Shaefer and Edin 2012: 2). During the same period, the number of children living in extremely poor households rose from 1.4 million to 2.8 million (Shaefer and Edin 2012: 4). Importantly, the study notes that there is a connection between the growth in extreme poverty and welfare reform: "The prevalence of extreme poverty rose sharply between 1996 and 2011. This growth has been concentrated among those groups that were most affected by the 1996 welfare reform" (Shaefer and Edin 2012: 4). In general, what welfare reform has meant is not the empowerment of the poor but their social and economic abandonment. Indeed, nowadays very few poor families qualify for or receive aid in the form of cash assistance, even in times of dire economic need. For example, as a result of a severe economic recession, the poverty rate in the United States jumped from 12.5 percent in 2007 to 15 percent in 2011 (Danziger, Chavez, and Cumberworth 2012: 1). However, in 2012, TANF benefits reached only 25 out of every 100 families in poverty (Floyd and Schott 2013: 1). By contrast, in 1979, 82 out of every 100 poor families received AFDC assistance (Trisi and Pavetti 2012: 1). This abandonment of the poor is consistent with neoliberalism as a political mentality that depoliticizes social problems—that treats poverty as the result of individual failings for which the state need bear no responsibility, rather than as a socially produced condition that requires governmental intervention.

Under neoliberalism, then, the impoverished and dispossessed of American society, who are often racial minorities, have generally been relegated to spaces of disposability (Giroux 2006, 2008). Indeed, Henry Giroux argues that as the welfare "state is displaced by the market, a new kind of politics is emerging in which some lives, if not whole groups, are seen as disposable and redundant" (2008: 594). So, whereas in the past marginalized populations could expect some support from the state, today they are generally left to fend for themselves. The state at present feels little compulsion to care for its underprivileged citizens, to take actions that mitigate their hardship and suffering. It has become so feeble with respect to social protection that vast numbers of individuals are being left without health care, education, housing, and retirement benefits (DiFazio 2006, Giroux 2006). In theory, the market is supposed to take the place of the state and provide for the population. However, although it might afford social protection to the rich and middle classes, it provides little security to the poor, the sick, the elderly, and the marginalized (Giroux 2006). Ultimately, in advancing a market-based ethic and in disavowing public policies that support life-sustaining social services, neoliberalism has led to the general immiseration of the American population. Indeed, for many the neoliberalization of life has meant the precarization of life.

Neoliberalism, BiDil, and Racialized Medicine

There is no doubt that BiDil and racialized medicine are by and large products of the contemporary neoliberal milieu. One of the areas in which the neoliberal emphasis on individual responsibility is most evident is health care (Galvin 2002, Crawford 2006, Rose 2007, Savard 2013). Under neoliberalism, a duty to be healthy and well has become a central element in the contemporary care of the self. "Lose weight!" "Eat right!" "Sleep well!" "Stop smoking!" "Drink responsibly!" "Practice safe sex!" "Just say no to drugs!" Such are the popular injunctions to be healthy that we hear today. This duty to be well is an ideology that sociologists have come to describe as *healthism*. According to Robert Crawford,

> [healthism] is defined ... as the preoccupation with personal health as a primary—often *the* primary—focus for the definition and achievement of well-being; a goal which is to be attained primarily through the modification of life styles, with or without therapeutic help. The etiology of disease may be seen as complex, but healthism treats individual behavior, attitudes, and emotions as relevant symptoms needing attention. Healthism will acknowledge, in other words, that health problems may originate outside the individual, e.g. in the American diet, but since these problems are also behavioral, solutions are seen to lie within the realm of individual choice. Hence, they require above all else the assumption of individual responsibility. [1980: 368]

Healthism, in other words, takes the pursuit of good health to be a necessary part of a person's welfare. Moreover, it posits that the upkeep of such a state of health is the responsibility of the individual, insisting that human beings can and should develop the personal capacity to prevent illness (Greco 1993). A key aspect of healthism is thus the expectation that individuals will adopt a calculative and prudent disposition toward health risks and insecurities, that they will police their own behavior in such a way as to minimize their exposure to health dangers and thereby maximize their life and well-being.

Not surprisingly, the principle mechanism through which people are expected to insure and ensure their health is not the state but the market In a neoliberal context, striving after a healthy existence has come to depend on consuming a range of goods and services, not only medical care proper but also a host of products that are marketed for their health-fostering properties: exercise machines, individualized fitness programs, weight loss centers, nutritious foods, and so forth (Petersen and Lupton 1996). Indeed, taking proper care of oneself nowadays means purchasing health and happiness in the marketplace. However, not everyone has the financial resources to be a proper, self-caring neoliberal subject. In 2012, for example, about 15.4 percent of the US population had no health insurance (DeNavas-Walt, Proctor, and Smith 2013: 22). These uninsured were generally poor people who could not afford to buy private health insurance and were not provided health care by the state (Seccombe and Hoffman 2007).[2] The rate of uninsurance was particularly high among poor racial minorities. In 2012, the rate for African Americans was 19.0 percent and for Latinos it was 29.1 percent (DeNavas-Walt, Proctor, and Smith 2013: 26). Insurance is important in the United States because it is the primary mechanism by which individuals and families access the health care system. Compared to people with insurance, the uninsured utilize the health

2 In 2012, about a quarter of all individuals in households earning less than $25,000 per year had no health insurance (DeNavas-Walt, Proctor, and Smith 2013: 28).

care system less frequently, depend more on emergency rooms for their care, are not as likely to have a reliable source of medical treatment, suffer more from a range of acute and chronic illnesses, and are generally more exposed to pain, distress, and death (Seccombe and Hoffman 2007). Health insurance, then, is a critical source of security to which millions of poor people, especially racial minorities, have little or no access, the consequence being the impoverishment of their health and well-being.[3]

Both BiDil and racialized medicine in general very much reflect healthism's emphasis on personal responsibility and market fundamentalism. Let us take BiDil first. As noted in Chapter 3, BiDil is deeply linked to questions of vital rights. The existence of the drug is about the entitlement of African Americans to the benefits of modern medicine. However, the rights connected to BiDil are not generally social rights but neoliberal ones. Indeed, the main demand that BiDil's advocates placed on the state was for the FDA to approve the drug so that it could be made available in the marketplace. Such a demand is a consumerist rather than a social one. The state was not asked to be a purveyor of health care. Rather, it was simply expected to create the conditions for bringing a drug product to market. In this context, BiDil represents a call to African Americans to take responsibility for their health by purchasing and consuming the drug (Krupar and Ehlers forthcoming). On the patient education website for BiDil, African Americans are told, "When it comes to heart failure, your doctor can do a lot of things to help and support you. But you—the patient—are in the driver's seat. Your choices and actions can make a difference in how well you manage your heart failure symptoms" (Arbor Pharmaceuticals 2012). One of the choices that African American patients are implicitly expected to make is to ask their doctors to prescribe BiDil to them. The neoliberal emphasis on the duty to be well is clearly in evidence here. African American patients are essentially exhorted to be active and responsible consumers of medical products and services. They are expected to be knowledgeable about their conditions and to turn to the market to obtain treatment and generate health. They are thus imagined as active patient-consumers who take upon themselves the principal responsibility for administering their own health.

As it turns out, very few African Americans who could benefit from BiDil have been prescribed the drug (Washington Legal Foundation 2008, Roberts 2011b, Pollock 2012). As noted in Chapter 5, because of the high price of

3 The Patient Protection and Affordable Care Act, an Obama administration initiative that was signed into law in 2010, is supposed to extend health insurance coverage to millions of uninsured Americans. However, an analysis of census data by *The New York Times* shows that the law will leave out "two-thirds of the poor blacks and single mothers and more than half of the low-wage workers who do not have insurance" (Tavernise and Gebeloff 2013).

BiDil and the availability of less expensive generic alternatives, many private health insurance plans have opted not to cover the drug, and those that do cover it generally require high monthly copayments (Rusert and Royal 2011). Government-sponsored health plans have also failed to cover the drug. For example, the Centers for Medicare and Medicaid Services (CMS)—the US federal agency that administers Medicare, Medicaid, and the Children's Health Insurance Program—does not require Medicare Part D plans to reimburse patients for BiDil (Roberts 2011b).[4] The reluctance of both private and government insurance plans to cover BiDil means that a significant portion of the potential African American heart failure population—about 70 percent of those over the age of 45—lack health insurance coverage for the drug or are required to pay hefty insurance copayments (Westphal 2006). So, after all the work that went into convincing the FDA to approve BiDil, with arguments about the need to reduce health disparities and alleviate black suffering, the drug failed to reach its market. A drug that was presumably produced to foster the lives of African Americans is thus not readily available to this population (Krupar and Ehlers forthcoming). This failure of BiDil to reach African Americans reflects a neoliberal milieu in which the state has generally ceased to provide social protection to its population and in which the market works only for those who have the ability to pay. It speaks to the corporal abandonment under neoliberalism of people who lack the financial wherewithal to purchase the medical and other goods necessary to achieve proper health (Roberts 2011b).

I should note that NitroMed did develop a patient assistance program for people who could not afford treatment with BiDil (NitroMed 2007e). Called NitroMed Cares, the program helped uninsured patients obtain free supplies of the drug and assisted insured patients in covering copayments for their prescriptions. Although it was no doubt a charitable practice, NitroMed's assistance program needs to be understood as part of the company's pricing

---

4 According to the Washington Legal Foundation (2008), CMS insists that instead of heart failure patients being provided with BiDil, they should be prescribed the cheaper generic alternatives: ISDN (isosorbide dinitrate) and HYD (hydralazine hydrochloride). However, the Foundation argues that, "for a variety of reasons, doctors are reluctant to adopt CMS's proposed generic substitute. Those reasons include: (1) ISDN and HYD are not available in prescription sizes that match the fixed-dose combination offered in BiDil—the only combination determined to be effective in clinical trials; (2) because neither ISDN nor HYD is approved for treatment of heart failure, there is no labeling available to guide doctors in making such prescriptions; and (3) asking patients to take many more pills each day substantially increases the likelihood that patients will not comply with treatment regimens" (Washington Legal Foundation 2008). Because doctors are unwilling to prescribe the generic alternative, few African Americans are benefiting from the hydralazine/isosorbide dinitrate combination in any form (Pollock 2012).

and profit-generating strategy (Pollock 2012). In his analysis of Novartis's anti-cancer drug Glivec, Stefan Ecks (2008) notes that pharmaceutical companies nowadays routinely give populations in need free access to their products. What this practice does is allow companies to present themselves as good corporate citizens. They then use the ethical credibility that this image gives them to sell the drug at high prices to those who can afford to pay. In the case of Glivec, Novatis donates the drug in resource-poor places such as India so that it can charge a premium for the medication in the wealthier North American and European markets. The practice of providing the poor with free drugs is thus ultimately about producing wealth. I suggest that this is precisely the case with respect to BiDil. Through NitroMed Cares, NitroMed clearly presented itself as a benevolent entity concerned with the health of poor African Americans. However, one can argue that the company gave away BiDil for free to the poor only so that it could gain the moral authority necessary to charge high prices to, and therefore generate profits from, people with the resources to purchase the drug. So, although NitroMed might not have abandoned African Americans, the company undoubtedly sought to foster the lives of poor blacks only because there was a potential for financial gain.[5]

A neoliberal ethos is also very much at work with respect to racialized medicine more broadly. As noted in Chapter 4, genetic researchers generally have a complex, nonreductionist take on race and genetics. For example, although they have certainly highlighted the genetic nature of heart failure in African Americans, they have not minimized social and environmental determinants. In fact, they have argued that factors such as poor access to good health care services and exposure to environmental pollutants contribute to high heart failure rates among blacks. However, when socio-environmental factors are taken into account in genetic medicine, race-based medicine included, they are often treated simply as triggers—as sparks that activate molecular changes in an individual's body. Disease is thus seen as fundamentally a problem of the body. It is how the body responds to exogenous stimuli, and not necessarily the stimuli themselves, that is important. The key to producing health is therefore knowledge of the body and its genetic processes. This knowledge allows researchers to devise medical technologies designed to prevent, resolve, or alleviate the body's maladies. In a neoliberal context,

5 Ultimately, NitroMed Cares did not succeed in ensuring access to the drug for poor blacks. As Anne Pollock (2012) argues, a basic problem with NitroMed's drug donation effort was that it underestimated just how medically underserved the African American population is. She notes, "Since BiDil's patient population is already often underserved by overstretched doctors, it is unrealistic to expect those doctors to take the uncompensated time to do the paperwork necessary to get patients the free drugs" (166).

such a model of well-being has intrinsic appeal. If it is possible to remediate illness through molecular medical interventions, then there is no need for the state to deal with social inequalities, environmental pollutants, and other factors that contribute to the production of poor health. Genetic medicine can thus be used by the state as a pretext to absolve itself of the responsibility for social investment in the population and to make health a matter of only personal responsibility, something to be procured through purchasing genetic products in the marketplace. For neoliberalism, then, the appeal of genetic medicine is that it promises to produce both health and wealth (because biomedical technologies present opportunities for capitalization), all without the necessity of costly social interventions (Nadesan 2013).

It is already evident that the characterization of diseases as genetic, even where it is clear that social factors are involved, has ushered in a trend to address maladies through biomedical interventions (genetic screening, genetically tailored therapy, and so forth) rather than by ameliorating conditions in the social environment (Roberts 2011a). A case in point is autism. Nowadays autism is largely regarded as a genetic condition, even though research suggests a strong role for environmental pollutants (for example, lead, mercury, ionizing radiation, industrial chemicals, and pesticides) in producing the disorder (Lauritsen and Ewald 2001, Nadesan 2013). A primary goal of autism research has thus become to find genes for autism, the ultimate goal being to develop pharmaceuticals and other commercial technologies to manage the condition. The problem with putting research emphasis on the genetics of autism, as Majia Holmer Nadesan points out, is that

> the seductive combination of genes and dollars has the potential to crowd out other research trajectories and autism-funding priorities. The concern here is that knowledge and products developed by the pharmaceutical-research complex will likely promote autism detection (tests) and pharmaceutical "management" over the more costly (in terms of initial investments) therapeutic approaches that are labor- and resource-intensive (such as sensory-integration therapy and special education services) and over alternative research approaches that might curtail industry profits by foregrounding environmental explanations for autism and other syndromes and diseases. [2013: 123]

This scenario, that other autism funding priorities will be crowded out, appears to have become reality in the United States. Today, little federal funding exists for environmental research on autism (Nadesan 2013), so autism prevention efforts that emphasize environmental solutions, as opposed to pharmaceutical cures, are practically nonexistent. Furthermore, at the national level, there is almost no public funding for services to help individuals diagnosed with autism to live meaningful lives. The framing of autism as a genetic disorder is thus leading to a minimization of the need to attend to the social environment as a way of preventing and managing autism. In the process, the state is absolved of the responsibility for monitoring industry and regulating contaminants known to contribute to the production of developmental disorders (Nadesan 2013).

Given the increased tendency to deal with diseases marked as genetic strictly through technical means, the rise of race-based medicine portends a similar trend with respect to how the maladies of racialized populations are managed. Despite the proven role of social factors such as racial discrimination and poverty in explaining racial disparities in health, the suggestion that genetic research holds promise in the campaign against such inequalities finds fertile ground in a neoliberal milieu (Sankar et al. 2004). The characterization of racial health disparities in terms of genetics essentially means that the state does not have to act to address environmental factors in order to produce health. Rather, it can simply let the market handle socially produced health problems through the manufacture of racially targeted medications and other technologies for mass consumption. Thus, as Dorothy Roberts argues,

> racial medicine has tremendous potential to affect the direction of state efforts to address health disparities, and racial inequality more broadly, by diverting attention from the structural causes of racial inequities toward genetic explanations and technological solutions. The public may think that race-based medicine shifts responsibility for addressing disease from the government to the individual by suggesting that health disparities are a result of genetic variation rather than inequitable social structures and access to health care. [2011a: 542]

Given years of retrenchment, the state has already reduced support for social programs meant to cultivate the life and welfare of disadvantaged populations, including racialized minorities. The suggestion that the problem of health disparities can be resolved through racial medicine only gives more ammunition to the neoliberal project of social disinvestment. Instead of fostering racial life, then, race-based medicine will likely make it more precarious. Indeed, to the extent that racialized medicine compels continued disinvestment in social programs, the effect will be to further impoverish the lives and health of racial minority populations.

Conclusion

In this concluding chapter, I have argued that as political government has progressively abandoned its role as social protector of the population, individuals in the United States have been left with the responsibility of securing their own lives against the vagaries of social and economic existence. The result of this neoliberalization of life has been to make living exceedingly precarious for marginalized populations in American society. The promotion of racial medicine as a way to resolve the problem of health disparities will likely only exacerbate this abandonment. BiDil certainly saves lives, but the net effect of investing in racialized medicine, if it is at the expense of social programming, will be to diminish racial life. There is no doubt that genetics has an impact upon practically all facets of health. However, a large body of research suggests that the contribution of genetics to patterns of health disparity in the United States is minor in comparison to social and environmental factors (Sankar et al. 2004, Brooks and King 2008). Health disparities are thus not principally a matter of genetics. Rather, they are about the biological materialization of social inequality (Braun 2002, Krieger and Smith 2004). They point to how the historical weight of poverty and exclusion makes racial minority populations susceptible to suffering from acute illness, chronic disease, social epidemics, and so forth (Brooks and King 2008). The way to remedy the problem of health inequality is thus not through racial therapeutics, which burden individuals with alleviating their own unequal health statuses, but through universalizing access to health care, investing in minority neighborhoods, improving the education system, curbing poverty, and eliminating racial discrimination (Brooks and King 2008, Roberts 2011a). Ultimately, racial health rests on the willingness of the state to invest in and take care of its marginal populations.

Bibliography

Abramovitz, M. 2000. *Under Attack: Fighting Back*. New York: Monthly Review Press.

Abu El-Haj, N. 2007. The genetic reinscription of race. *Annual Review of Anthropology*, 36, 283–300.

Acs, G. and Loprest, P. 2004a. Leaving welfare: challenges in a new economy. *Employment Research Newsletter*, 11(4), 5–6.

Acs, G. and Loprest, P. 2004b. *Leaving Welfare: Employment and Well-Being of Families that Left Welfare in the Post-Entitlement Era*. Kalamazoo, MI: W.E. Upjohn Institute of Employment Research.

Agamben, G. 1998. *Homo Sacer: Sovereign Power and Bare Life*. Stanford, CA: Stanford University Press.

Alcon. 2003. Travatan® Project Focus enjoys success as it brings free glaucoma screenings to at-risk African Americans. Alcon press release, July 21. [Online]. Available at: http://invest.alconinc.com/phoenix.zhtml?c=130946&p=irol-newsArticle_print&ID=433049&highlight [accessed: September 26, 2013].

Alcon. 2013. *Travatan Z®: Highlights of Prescribing Information*. Fort Worth, TX: Alcon Laboratories.

Amin, A. (ed.). 1994. *Post-Fordism: A Reader*. Malden, MA: Wiley-Blackwell.

Arbor Pharmaceuticals. 2012. What you can do. [Online]. Available at: http://www.bidil.com/pnt/do.php [accessed: November 26, 2013].

Association of Black Cardiologists (ABC) and National Institutes of Health (NIH). 2004. *Eliminating Disparities in Cardiovascular Care and Outcomes: Roadmap to 2010*. Atlanta, GA and Bethesda, MD: Association of Black Cardiologists and National Institutes of Health.

Association of Black Cardiologists (ABC) and NitroMed. n.d. *7 Steps to a Healthy Heart*. Atlanta, GA and Lexington, MA: ABC and NitroMed.

AstraZeneca. 2013. *Crestor: Highlights of Prescribing Information*. Wilmington, DE: AstraZeneca Pharmaceuticals.

Bailey, P. and Jones, A. 2012. Want to educate minorities? Share their voice. *Multicultural Health Marketing*, 1, 14–15.

Barbot, J. 2006. How to build an "active" patient? The work of AIDS associations in France. *Social Science and Medicine*, 62(3), 538–51.

Bauman, Z. 1989. *Modernity and the Holocaust*. Ithaca, NY: Cornell University Press.

Berrick, J.D. 2001. Targeting social welfare in the United States: personal responsibility, private behavior, and public benefits, in *Targeting Social Benefits: International Perspectives and Trends*, edited by N. Gilbert. New Brunswick, NJ: Transaction, 129–56.

Bibbins-Domingo, K. and Fernandez, A. 2007. BiDil for heart failure in black patients: implications of the US Food and Drug Administration approval. *Annals of Internal Medicine*, 146(1), 52–6.

Biehl, J. 2007. *Will to Live: AIDS Therapies and the Politics of Survival*. Princeton, NJ: Princeton University Press.

Black Issues in Higher Education. 2002. Heart failure in blacks may signal a "different disease." *Black Issues in Higher Education*, 19(9), 26–7.

Bliss, C. 2012. *Race Decoded: The Genomic Fight for Social Justice*. Stanford, CA: Stanford University Press.

Bloche, G.M. 2004. Race-based therapeutics. *New England Journal of Medicine*, 351, 2035–7.

Blumenbach, J.F. 1969. *On the Natural Varieties of Mankind*. New York: Bergman.

Brandt, A.M. 1978. Racism and research: the case of the Tuskegee Syphilis Study. *The Hastings Center Report*, 8(6), 21–9.

Braun, L. 2002. Race, ethnicity, and health: can genetics explain disparities? *Perspectives in Biology and Medicine*, 45(2), 159–74.

Braun, L. 2006. Reifying human difference: the debate on genetics, race, and health. *International Journal of Health Services*, 36(3), 557–73.

Briggs, C.L. and Hallin, D.C. 2007. Biocommunicability: the neoliberal subject and its contradictions in news coverage of health issues. *Social Text*, 25(4), 43–66.

Bristol-Myers Squibb. 2011. *Coumadin: Highlights of Prescribing Information*. Princeton, NJ: Bristol-Myers Squibb.

Brody, H. and Hunt, L.M. 2006. BiDil: assessing a race-based pharmaceutical. *Annals of Family Medicine*, 4(6), 556–60.

Brooks, J.D. and King, M.L. 2008. *Geneticizing Disease: Implications for Racial Health Disparities*. Washington, DC: Center for American Progress.

Brown, N.J., Ray, W.A., Snowden, M. and Griffin, M.R. 1996. Black Americans have an increased rate of angiotensin converting enzyme inhibitor-associated angioedema. *Clinical Pharmacology & Therapeutics*, 60(1), 8–13.

Brown, W. 2003. Neo-liberalism and the end of liberal democracy. *Theory and Event*, 7(1). [Online]. Available at: http://muse.jhu.edu/journals/theory_and_event/v007/7.1brown.html [accessed: December 11, 2013].

Brown, W. 2006. American nightmare: neoliberalism, neoconvervatism, and de-democratization. *Political Theory*, 34(2), 690–714.

Budnitz, D.S., Lovegrove, M.C., Shehab, N. and Richards, C.L. 2011. Emergency hospitalizations for adverse drug events in older Americans. *New England Journal of Medicine*, 365(21), 2002–12.

Burchard, E.G., Ziv, E., Coyle, N., Gomez, S.L., Tang, H., Karter, A.J. et al. 2003. The importance of race and ethnic background in biomedical research and clinical practice. *New England Journal of Medicine*, 348(12), 1170–75.

Business Wire. 2007. NAACP-New England area conference commends Prescription Pathway^{SM} Medicare prescription drug plan on availability of BiDil® for plan members. [Online]. Available at: http://investor.uafc.com/phoenix.zhtml?c=75985&p=irol-newsArticle&ID=952330&highlight [accessed: March 22, 2008].

Butler, J. 2004. *Precarious Life: The Powers of Mourning and Violence.* New York: Verso.

Butrick, M., Roter, D., Kaphingst, K., Erby, L.H., Harywood Jr., C., Beach, M.C. et al. 2011. Patient reactions to personalized medicine vignettes: an experimental design. *Genetics in Medicine*, 13(5), 421–8.

Calavita, K. 1996. The new politics of immigration: "balanced-budget conservatism" and the symbolism of Proposition 187. *Social Problems*, 43(3), 284–305.

Calavita, K. 1998. Immigration, law, and marginalization in a global economy: notes from Spain. *Law & Society Review*, 32(3), 529–66.

Carson, P., Ziesche, S., Johnson, G. and Cohn, J.N. 1999. Racial differences in response to therapy for heart failure: analysis of the Vasodilator-Heart Failure Trials. *Journal of Cardiac Failure*, 5(3), 178–87.

Castel, R. 1999. *Les métamorphoses de la question sociale.* Paris: Gallimard.

Cepeda, M.S., Farrar, J.T., Roa, J.H., Boston, R., Meng, Q.C., Ruiz, F. et al. 2001. Ethnicity influences morphine pharmacokinetics and pharmacodynamics. *Clinical Pharmacology and Therapeutics*, 70(4), 351–61.

Christensen, D.M. 2005. Testimony, in *Cardiovascular and Renal Drugs Advisory Committee.* Vol. 2. Center for Drug Evaluation and Research, US Food and Drug Administration. Washington, DC: US Department of Health and Human Services, 203–10.

Clarke, A.E., Shim, J.K., Mamo, L., Fosket, J.R. and Fishman, J.R. 2010. Biomedicalization: technoscientific transformations of health, illness, and US biomedicine, in *Biomedicalization: Technoscience, Health, and Illness in the US*, edited by A.E. Clarke, L. Mamo, J.R. Fosket, J.R. Fishman and J.K. Shim. Durham, NC: Duke University Press, 47–87.

Clark-Hitt, R., Malat, J., Burgess, D. and Friedemann-Sanchez, G. 2010. Doctors' and nurses' explanations for racial disparities in medical treatment. *Journal of Health Care for the Poor and Underserved*, 21(1), 386–400.

Clinton, W.J. 1993. *Address Before a Joint Session of Congress on Administration Goals.* February 17. [Online]. Available at: http://www.presidency.ucsb.edu/ws/?pid=47232 [accessed: December 10, 2013].

Cohn, J.N. 1973. Vasodilator therapy for heart failure: the influence of impedance on left ventricular performance. *Circulation*, 48, 5–8.

Cohn, J.N. 1987. Method of reducing mortality associated with congestive heart failure using hydralazine and isosorbide dinitrate. US Patent 4,868,179, filed April 22, 1987.

Cohn, J.N. 1993. Introduction. *Circulation*, 87(6), VI-1–VI-4.

Cohn, J.N. 2003. Discussion. *Journal of Cardiac Failure*, 9(5), S205–S209.

Cohn, J.N. 2005. A-HeFT: old dog, new endothelial tricks. *Current Issues in Cardiology*, 32(3), 366–8.

Cohn, J.N., Archibald, D.G., Ziesche, S., Franciosa, J.A., Harston, W.E., Tristani, F.E. et al. 1986. Effect of vasodilator therapy on mortality in chronic congestive heart failure: results of a Veterans Administration Cooperative Study. *New England Journal of Medicine*, 314(24), 1547–52.

Cohn, J.N. and Carson, J. 2000. Methods of treating and preventing congestive heart failure with hydralazine compounds and isosorbide dinitrate or isosorbide mononitrate. US Patent 6,465,463, filed September 8.

Cohn, J.N., Johnson, G., Ziesche, S., Cobb, F., Francis, G., Tristani, F. et al. 1991. A comparison of enalapril with hydralazine-isosorbide dinitrate in the treatment of chronic congestive heart failure. *New England Journal of Medicine*, 325(5), 303–10.

Collier, S.J. 2011. *Post-Soviet Social: Neoliberalism, Social Modernity, Biopolitics*. Princeton, NJ: Princeton University Press.

Collins, F.S., Green, E.D., Guttmacher, A.E. and Guyer, M.S., on behalf of the US National Human Genome Research Institute. 2003. A vision for the future of genomics research: a blueprint for the genomic era. *Nature*, 422, 835–47.

Condit, C., Templeton, A., Bates, B.R., Bevan, J.L and Harris, T.M. 2003. Attitudinal barriers to delivery of race-targeted pharmacogenomics among informed lay persons. *Genetics in Medicine*, 5(5), 385–92.

Cooper, M. 2008. *Life as Surplus: Biotechnology and Capitalism in the Neoliberal Era*. Seattle: University of Washington Press.

Cooper, R.S. 2004. Genetic factors in ethnic disparities in health, in *Critical Perspectives on Racial and Ethnic Differences in Health in Late Life*, edited by N.B. Anderson, R.A. Bulatao and B. Cohen. Washington, DC: National Academies Press, 269–309.

Crawford, R. 1980. Healthism and the medicalization of everyday life. *International Journal of Health Services*, 10(3), 365–88.

Crawford, R. 2006. Health as a meaningful social practice. *Health: An Interdisciplinary Journal for the Social Study of Health, Illness, and Medicine*, 10(4), 401–20.

Curry, C. 2005. Testimony, in *Cardiovascular and Renal Drugs Advisory Committee*. Vol. 2. Center for Drug Evaluation and Research, US Food and Drug Administration. Washington, DC: US Department of Health and Human Services, 229–34.

Danziger, S., Chavez, K. and Cumberworth, E. 2012. *Poverty and the Great Recession*. Stanford, CA: Stanford Center on Poverty and Inequality.

Dean, M. 1999. *Governmentality: Power and Rule in Modern Society*. London: Sage.

De Marco, M. 2010. Views on personalized medicine: do the attitudes of African American and white prescription drug consumers differ? *Public Health Genomics*, 13, 276–83.

De Maria, N., Colantoni, A., Idilman, R., Friedlander, L., Harig, J. and Van Thiel, D.H. 2002. Impaired response to high-dose interferon treatment in African-Americans with chronic hepatitis C. *Hepatogastroenterology*, 49(45), 788–92.

DeNavas-Walt, C., Proctor, B.D. and Smith, J.C. 2013. *Income, Poverty, and Health Insurance Coverage in the United States: 2012*. Washington, DC: US Census Bureau.

DiFazio, W. 2006. Katrina and President George W. Bush forever. *Situations*, 1(2), 87–92.

Downey, L.J. 2012. BiDil: alive and kicking. *Lancet*, 379, 1876.

Duncan, J.S. 2007. *In the Shadows of the Tropics: Climate, Race, and Biopower in Nineteenth Century Ceylon*. Burlington, VT: Ashgate.

Duster, T. 2006. The molecular reinscription of race: unanticipated issues in biotechnology and forensic science. *Patterns of Prejudice*, 40(4–5), 427–41.

Duster, T. 2007. Medicalisation of race. *Lancet*, 369, 702–4.

Ecks, S. 2008. Global pharmaceutical markets and corporate citizenship: the case of Novartis' anti-cancer drug Glivec. *Biosocieties*, 3(2), 165–81.

Ellison, G.T.H., Kaufman, J.S., Head, R.F., Martin, P.A. and Kahn, J.D. 2008. Flaws in the US Food and Drug Administration's rationale for supporting the development and approval of BiDil as a treatment for heart failure only in black patients. *Journal of Law, Medicine & Ethics*, 36(3), 449–57.

Elsevier Business Intelligence. 2011. Arbor Pharmaceuticals acquires NitroMed. [Online]. Available at: http://www.elsevierbi.com/deals/201110215 [accessed: October 10, 2013].

Epstein, S. 2007. *Inclusion: The Politics of Difference in Medical Research*. Chicago: University of Chicago Press.

Epstein, S. 2010. Beyond inclusion, beyond difference: the biopolitics of health, in *What's the Use of Race? Modern Governance and the Biology of Difference*, edited by I. Whitmarsh and D.S. Jones. Cambridge, MA: MIT Press, 63–87.

Exner, D.V., Dries, D.L., Domanski, M. and Cohn, J.N. 2001. Lesser response to angiotensin-converting-enzyme inhibitor therapy in black as compared to white patients with left ventricular dysfunction. *New England Journal of Medicine*, 344(18), 1351–7.

Fassin, D. 2001. The biopolitics of otherness: undocumented foreigners and racial discrimination in French public debate. *Anthropology Today*, 17(1), 3–7.

Fassin, D. 2007. Humanitarianism as a politics of life. *Public Culture*, 19(3), 499–520.

Fausto-Sterling, A. 2004. Refashioning race: DNA and the politics of health care. *Differences: A Journal of Feminist Cultural Studies*, 15(3), 1–37.

FD (Fair Disclosure) Wire. 2004. NitroMed, Inc. at Deutsche Bank Securities 29th Annual Health Care Conference. [Online]. Available at: http://www.accessmylibrary.com/coms2/summary_0286-1420302_ITM [accessed: May 30, 2013].

Ferdinand, K.C. 2006a. Improving care for African-American heart failure patients. *US Cardiovascular Disease*, 3(1), 86–9.

Ferdinand, K.C. 2006b. The isosorbide-hydralazine story: is there a case for race-based cardiovascular medicine? *Journal of Clinical Hypertension*, 8(3), 156–8.

Fisher, J.A. 2009. *Medical Research for Hire: The Political Economy of Pharmaceutical Clinical Trials*. New Brunswick, NJ: Rutgers University Press.

Floyd, I. and Schott, L. 2013. *TNAF Cash Benefits Continued to Lose Value in 2013*. Washington, DC: Center on Budget and Policy Priorities.

Food and Drug Administration Modernization Act (FDAMA) of 1997. Public Law 105–115 [S. 830]. 105th Congress, November 21.

Forest Laboratories. 2007. Nebivolol lowers blood pressure in African Americans with stage I-II hypertension as demonstrated in a study published in the Journal of Clinical Hypertension. Forest Laboratories press release, November 1. [Online]. Available at: http://investor.frx.com/press-release/rd-news/update-nebivolol-lowers-blood-pressure-african-americans-stage-i-ii-hypertensi [accessed: October 10, 2013].

Forest Laboratories. 2011. *Bystolic: Highlights of Prescribing Information*. St. Louis, MO: Forest Laboratories.

Foucault, M. 1980. *The History of Sexuality. Vol. 1: An Introduction*. New York: Vintage Books.

Foucault, M. 2000. Governmentality, in *The Essential Works of Foucault, 1954–1984. Vol. 3: Power*, edited by J.D. Faubion. New York: New Press, 201–22.

Foucault, M. 2003. 17 March 1976, in *Society Must Be Defended: Lectures at the Collège de France, 1975–1976*. New York: Picador, 239–64.

Frank, D., Gallagher, T.H., Sellers, S.L., Cooper, L.A., Price, E.G., Odunlami, A.O. et al. 2010. Primary care physicians' attitudes regarding race-based therapies. *Journal of General Internal Medicine*, 25(5), 384–9.

Frank, R. 2001. A reconceptualization of the role of biology in contributing to race/ethnic disparities in health outcomes. *Population Research and Policy Review*, 20(6), 441–55.

Franklin, S. 2000. Life itself: global nature and the genetic imaginary, in *Global Nature, Global Culture*, edited by S. Franklin, C. Lury and J. Stacey. London: Sage, 188–227.

Fraser, N. 1993. Clintonism, welfare, and the antisocial wage: the emergence of a neoliberal political imaginary. *Rethinking Marxism*, 6(1), 9–23.

Fujimura, J.H., Duster, T. and Rajagopalan, R. 2008. Introduction: race, genetics, and disease: questions of evidence, matters of consequence. *Social Studies of Science*, 38(5), 643–56.

Fullwiley, D. 2004. From discriminate biopower to everyday biopolitics: views on sickle cell testing in Dakar. *Medical Anthropology*, 23(2), 157–94.

Fullwiley, D. 2007. The molecularization of race: institutionalizing human difference in pharmacogenetics practice. *Sciences as Culture*, 16(1), 1–30.

Fullwiley, D. 2011. *The Enculturated Gene: Sickle Cell Health Politics and Biological Difference in West Africa*. Princeton, NJ: Princeton University Press.

Galvin, R. 2002. Disturbing notions of chronic illness and individual responsibility: towards a genealogy of morals. *Health: An Interdisciplinary Journal for the Social Study of Health, Illness, and Medicine*, 6(2), 107–37.

Gellene, D. 2005. Heart pill intended only for blacks sparks debate. *Los Angeles Times*, June 16. [Online]. Available at: http://articles.latimes.com/2005/jun/16/business/fi-bidil16 [accessed: October 9, 2013].

Giacomini, K.M., Brett, C.M., Altman, R.B., Benowitz, N.L., Dolan, M.E., Flockhart, D.A. et al., for the Pharmacogenetics Research Network. 2007. The Pharmacogenetics Research Network: from SNP discovery to clinical drug response. *Clinical Pharmacology & Therapeutics*, 81(1), 328–45.

Gibbon, S. and Novas, C. (eds). 2008. *Biosocialities, Genetics and the Social Sciences: Making Biologies and Identities*. London: Routledge.

Gibbs, C.R., Beevers, D.G. and Lip, G.Y.H. 1999. The management of hypertensive disease in black patients. *QJM: An International Journal of Medicine*, 92(4), 187–92.

Giroux, H.A. 2006. Reading Hurricane Katrina: race, class, and the biopolitics of disposability. *College Literature*, 33(3), 171–96.

Giroux, H.A. 2008. Beyond the biopolitics of disposability: rethinking neoliberalism in the new Gilded Age. *Social Identities*, 14(5), 587–620.

Goodman, A.H., Moses, Y.T. and Jones, J.L. 2012. *Race: Are We So Different?* Malden, MA: Wiley-Blackwell.

Gottweis, H., Salter, B. and Waldby, C. 2009. *The Global Politics of Human Embryonic Stem Cell Science: Regenerative Medicine in Transition*. New York: Palgrave Macmillan.

Greco, M. 1993. Psychosomatic subjects and the "duty to be well": personal agency within medical rationality. *Economy and Society*, 22(3), 357–72.

Guiha, N.H., Cohn, J.N., Mikulic, E., Franciosa, J.A. and Limas, C.J. 1974. Treatment of refractory heart failure with infusion of nitroprusside. *New England Journal of Medicine*, 291(12), 587–92.

Guillemette, C., Millikan, R.C., Newman, B. and Housman, D.E. 2000. Genetic polymorphisms in uridine diphospho-glucuronosyltransferase 1A1 and association with breast cancer among African Americas. *Cancer Research*, 60(4), 950–56.

Hacking, I. 1986. Making up people, in *Reconstructing Individualism: Autonomy, Individuality, and the Self in Western Thought*, edited by T.C. Heller, M. Sosna and D.E. Wellbery. Stanford, CA: Stanford University Press, 222–36.

Hamilton, J.A. 2008. Revitalizing difference in the HapMap: race and contemporary human genetic variation research. *Journal of Law, Medicine & Ethics*, 36(3), 471–7.

Happe, K.E. 2006. The rhetoric of race in breast cancer research. *Patterns of Prejudice*, 40(4–5), 461–80.

Happe, K.E. 2013. *The Material Gene: Gender, Race, and Heredity After the Human Genome Project*. New York: New York University Press.

Harrison, B. and Bluestone, B. 1988. *The Great U-Turn: Corporate Restructuring and the Polarizing of America*. New York: Basic Books.

Hartigan, J. (ed.). 2013. *Anthropology of Race: Genes, Biology, and Culture*. Santa Fe, NM: SAR Press.

Harvey, D. 1989. *The Condition of Postmodernity*. Oxford, UK: Basil Blackwell.

Harvey, D. 1991. Flexibility: threat or opportunity? *Socialist Review*, 21(1), 65–77.

Harvey, D. 2005. *A Brief History of Neoliberalism*. Oxford, UK: Oxford University Press.

Heart Failure Society of America (HSFA). n.d. *Quick Facts & Questions About Heart Failure*. [Online]. Available at: http://www.hfsa.org/heart_failure_facts.asp [accessed: July 3, 2008].

Hedgecoe, A. 2001. Schizophrenia and the narrative of enlightened geneticization. *Social Studies of Science*, 31(6), 875–911.

Hedgecoe, A. 2004. *The Politics of Personalised Medicine: Pharmacogenetics in the Clinic*. Cambridge, UK: Cambridge University Press.

Helgadottir, A., Hakonarson, H., Gulcher, J.R. and Gurney, M.E. 2010. Susceptibility gene for myocardial infarction, stroke, and PAOD: methods of treatment. US Patent 20100216863, filed August 26.

Hoffman, S. 2005. "Racially-tailored" medicine unraveled. *American University Law Review*, 55(2), 395–452.

Holmes, T.E. 2004. Vigilante awarded BiDil ad campaign. [Online]. Available at: http://www.docstoc.com/docs/40400345/Although-financial-terms-of-the-NitroMed-deal-were-not [accessed: October 10, 2013].

Humphreys, J.M. 2004. The multicultural economy 2004: America's minority buying power. *Georgia Business and Economic Conditions*, 64(3), 1–26.

Hung, H.M.J. 2005. *Statistical Review and Evaluation: BiDil*. Rockville, MD: US Food and Drug Administration.

Inda, J.X. 2006. *Targeting Immigrants: Government, Technology, and Ethics*. Malden, MA: Wiley-Blackwell.

Inda, J.X. 2007. The value of immigrant life, in *Women and Migration in the US–Mexico Borderlands*, edited by D.A. Segura and P. Zavella. Durham, NC: Duke University Press, 134–57.

Inda, J.X. 2011. Materializing hope: racial pharmaceuticals, suffering bodies, and biological citizenship, in *Corpus: An Interdisciplinary Reader on Bodies and Knowledge*, edited by M.J. Casper and P. Currah. New York: Palgrave Macmillan, 61–80.

Ishibe, N., Hankinson, S.E., Colditz, G.A., Spiegelman, D., Willett, W.C., Speizer, F.E. et al. 1998. Cigarette smoking, cytochrome P450 1A1 polymorphisms, and breast cancer risk in the Nurses' Health Study. *Cancer Research*, 58(4), 667–71.

Jackson Jr., J.P. and Weidman, N.M. 2006. *Race, Racism, and Science: Social Impact and Interaction*. New Brunswick, NJ: Rutgers University Press.

Jackson, R.L. 2001. Family welfare rolls show slight drop. *Los Angeles Times*, September 6, A14.

Jewell, M. 2006. Drug maker breaking new ground with grassroots marketing of BiDil. *Target Market News*, April 11. [Online]. Available at: http://targetmarketnews.com/storyid04170602.htm [accessed: March 8, 2008].

Johnmar, F. 2006. Conversations about race-based medicine: NitroMed's Michael L. Sabolinksi, M.D. Envisioning 2.0 Blog. [Online]. Retrieved from: http://fardj.prblogs.org/2006/06/27/conversations-about-race-based-medicine-nitromeds-michael-l-sabolinski-md [accessed: March 8, 2008].

Johnson, J.A. 2008. Ethnic differences in cardiovascular drug response: potential contribution of pharmacogenetics. *Circulation*, 118, 1383–93.

Jones, D.S. and Perlis, R.H. 2006. Pharmacogenetics, race, and psychiatry: prospects and challenges. *Harvard Review of Psychiatry*, 14(4), 92–108.

Jones, L.A. and Chilton, J.A. 2002. Impact of breast cancer on African American women: priority areas for research in the next decade. *American Journal of Public Health*, 92(4): 539–42.

Kahn, J. 2003. Getting the numbers right: statistical mischief and racial profiling in heart failure research. *Perspectives in Biology and Medicine*, 46(4), 473–83.

Kahn, J. 2004. How a drug becomes "ethnic": law, commerce, and the production of racial categories. *Yale Journal of Health Policy, Law, and Ethics*, 4(1), 1–46.

Kahn, J. 2005. From disparity to difference: how race-specific medicines may undermine policies to address inequalities in health care. *Southern California Interdisciplinary Law Journal*, 15, 105–29.

Kahn, J. 2009. Beyond BiDil: the expanding embrace of race in biomedical research and product development. *Saint Louis University Journal of Health Law & Policy*, 3(1), 61–92.

Kahn, J. 2013. *Race in a Bottle: The Story of BiDil and Racialized Medicine in a Post-Genomic Age*. New York: Columbia University Press.

Kalow, W. 2006. Pharmacogenetics and pharmacogenomics: origin, status, and the hope for personalized medicine. *Pharmacogenomics Journal*, 6, 162–5.

Kaufman, J.S., Nguyen, T.T. and Cooper, R.S. 2010. Race, medicine, and the science behind BiDil: how ACE-inhibition took the fall for the first ethnic drug. *The Review of Black Political Economy*, 37, 115–30.

Keita, S. 2005. Testimony, in *Cardiovascular and Renal Drugs Advisory Committee*. Vol. 2. Center for Drug Evaluation and Research, US Food and Drug Administration. Washington, DC: US Department of Health and Human Services, 221–4.

Kennedy, V.B. 2004. NitroMed soars on BiDil launch news. *MarketWatch*, August 2. [Online]. Available at: http://www.marketwatch.com/story/nitromed-soars-on-plans-for-cardiac-drugs-launch [accessed: October 10, 2013].

King, D. 1999. *In the Name of Liberalism: Illiberal Social Policy in the United States and Britain*. Oxford, UK: Oxford University Press.

Kittles, R.A. and Weiss, K.M. 2003. Race, ancestry, and genes: implications for defining disease risk. *Annual Review of Genomics and Human Genetics*, 4, 33–67.

Knight, K. 2005. The K Chronicles: "Bidil me this, blackman." [Online]. Available at: http://www.ibuzzle.com/editorials/6-27-2005-72179.asp [accessed: October 10, 2013].

Koenig, B.A., Lee, S.S.J. and Richardson, S.S. (eds). 2008. *Revisiting Race in a Genomic Age*. New Brunswick, NJ: Rutgers University Press.

Kreimer, S. 2007. BiDil not widely prescribed. *DOC News*, 4(7), 23. [Online]. Retrieved from: http://docnews.diabetesjournals.org/cgi/content/full/4/7/23 [accessed: February 2, 2008].

Krieger, N. 2002. Is breast cancer a disease of affluence, poverty, or both? The case of African American women. *American Journal of Public Health*, 92(4), 611–13.

Krieger, N. 2005. Stormy weather: race, gene expression, and the science of health disparities. *American Journal of Public Health*, 95(12), 2155–60.

Krieger, N. and Smith, G.D. 2004. "Bodies count," and body counts: social epidemiology and embodying inequality. *Epidemiologic Reviews*, 26(1), 92–103.

Krupar, S. and Ehlers, N. Forthcoming. Target: biomedicine and racialized geo-body-politics. *Occasion*.

Landzelius, K. 2006. Introduction: patient organization movements and new metamorphoses in patienthood. *Social Science & Medicine*, 62(3), 529–37.

Lauritsen, M.B. and Ewald, H. 2001. The genetics of autism. *Acta Psychiatrica Scandinavica*, 103(6), 411–27.

Lee, D. 2005. Testimony, in *Cardiovascular and Renal Drugs Advisory Committee*. Vol. 2. Center for Drug Evaluation and Research, US Food and Drug Administration. Washington, DC: US Department of Health and Human Services, 218–21.

Lee, S.S.J. 2006. Biobanks of a "racial kind": mining for difference in the new genetics. *Patterns of Prejudice*, 40(4–5), 443–60.

Lee, S.S.J., Mountain, J. and Koenig, B. 2001. The meaning of "race" in the new genomics: implications for health disparities research. *Yale Journal of Health Policy, Law, and Ethics*, 1(1), 33–75.

Lee, S.S.J., Mountain, J., Koenig, B., Altman, R., Brown, M., Camarillo, A. et al. 2008. The ethics of characterizing difference: guiding principles on using racial categories in human genetics. *Genome Biology*, 9(7), 404.1–404.4.

Lemtouni, S. 2005. *Clinical Review: BiDil*. Rockville, MD: US Food and Drug Administration.

Lombardo, P.A. and Dorr, G.M. 2006. Eugenics, medical education, and the Public Health Service: another perspective on the Tuskegee Syphilis Experiment. *Bulletin of the History of Medicine*, 80(2), 291–316.

Loprest, P. 2003. *Fewer Welfare Leavers Employed in Weak Economy*. Washington, DC: Urban Institute.

Malik, K. 2005. A colour coded prescription. [Online]. Available at: http://www.kenanmalik.com/tv/analysis_race%2Bmedicine.html [accessed: March 8, 2008].

Mamo, L. 2007. *Queering Reproduction: Achieving Pregnancy in the Age of Technoscience*. Durham, NC: Duke University Press.

Mbembe, A. 2003. Necropolitics. *Public Culture*, 15(1), 11–40.

McNair, L. 2010. HCV combination therapies. US Patent 20100226889, filed September 9.

McNamara, D.M., Tam, S.W., Sabolinski, M.L., Tobelmann, P., Janosko, K., Venkitachalam, L. et al. 2009. Endothelial nitric oxide synthase (NOS3) polymorphisms in African Americans with heart failure: results from the A-HeFT trial. *Journal of Cardiac Failure*, 15(3), 191–8.

Meadows, M. 2005. FDA approves heart drug for black patients. *FDA Consumer Magazine*, 39(5), 8–9.

Medco. 1991. *10-K*. [Online]. Available at: http://www.lexisnexis.com [accessed: July 24, 2008].

Medco. 1992. *Annual Report to Stockholders*. [Online]. Available at: http://www.lexisnexis.com [accessed: July 24, 2008].

Metzl, J.M. 2009. *The Protest Psychosis: How Schizophrenia Became a Black Disease*. Boston, MA: Beacon Press.

Meyer, U.A. 2004. Pharmacogenetics—five decades of therapeutic lessons from genetic diversity. *Nature Reviews Genetics*, 5, 669–76.

Miller, P. and Rose, N. 1990. Governing economic life. *Economy and Society*, 19(1), 1–31.

Mills, C. 2008. *The Philosophy of Agamben*. Montreal: McGill-Queen's University Press.

Mink, G. 1998. *Welfare's End*. Ithaca, NY: Cornell University Press.

Mol, A. 1998. Lived reality and the multiplicity of norms: a critical tribute to Georges Canguilhem. *Economy and Society*, 27(3–4), 274–84.

Montoya, M.J. 2011. *Making the Mexican Diabetic: Race, Science, and the Genetics of Inequality*. Berkeley: University of California Press.

Morning, A. 2011. *The Nature of Race: How Scientists Think and Teach About Human Difference*. Berkeley: University of California Press.

Moynihan, D.P. 1973. *The Politics of a Guaranteed Income: The Nixon Administration and the Family Assistance Plan*. New York: Random House.

Murray, C. 1984. *Losing Ground: American Social Policy, 1950–1980*. New York: Basic Books.

Nadesan, M.H. 2013. Autism and genetics: profit, risk, and bare life, in *Worlds of Autism: Across the Spectrum of Neurological Difference*, edited by J. Davidson and M. Orsini. Minneapolis: University of Minnesota Press, 117–42.

National Association for the Advancement of Colored People (NAACP). 2005a. *Emergency Resolution No. 7: BiDil in Treatment Plan of Black Patients with Congestive Heart Failure*. Baltimore, MD: NAACP.

National Association for the Advancement of Colored People (NAACP). 2005b. NAACP and NitroMed announce partnership to narrow disparities in cardiovascular health. *NAACP News*, December 14.

National Association for the Advancement of Colored People (NAACP). 2006. NAACP to help minority communities "Kick the Habit." *The NAACP Advocate*, 1(3), 3.

National Association for the Advancement of Colored People (NAACP). n.d. Health. [Online]. Available at: http://www.naacp.org/advocacy/health [accessed: March 22, 2008].

National Institute on Alcohol Abuse and Alcoholism (NIAAA). 2002. *Strategic Plan and Budget to Reduce and Ultimately Eliminate Health Disparities*. Bethesda, MD: US Department of Health and Human Services.

National Institutes of Health (NIH). 1994. *NIH Guidelines on the Inclusion of Women and Minorities as Subjects in Clinical Research*. [Online]. Available at: http://grants.nih.gov/grants/guide/notice-files/not94-100.html [accessed: September 25, 2012].

National Institutes of Health (NIH). 2002. *Strategic Research Plan and Budget to Reduce and Ultimately Eliminate Health Disparities. Vol. 1: Fiscal Years 2002–2006*. Bethesda, MD: US Department of Health and Human Services.

National Institutes of Health Revitalization Act (NIHRA) of 1993. Public Law 103–43 [S. 1]. 103rd Congress, June 10.

Neilson, B. 2006. Cultural studies and Giorgio Agamben, in *New Cultural Studies: Adventures in Theory*, edited by G. Hall and C. Birchall. Athens: University of Georgia Press, 128–45.

Nelson, A. 2012. *Body and Soul: The Black Panther Party and the Fight Against Medical Discrimination*. Minneapolis: University of Minnesota Press.

Nissen, S.E. 2005. Report from the Cardiovascular and Renal Drugs Advisory Committee, US Food and Drug Administration, July 15–16, 2005. *Circulation*, 112, 2043–6.

NitroMed. 2004. *Form 10-K*. Lexington, MA: NitroMed.

NitroMed. 2005a. *BiDil® (Isosorbide Dinitrate and Hydralazine Hydrochloride) Tables. NDA 20-727*. FDA Advisory Committee Briefing Document. Lexington, MA: NitroMed.

NitroMed. 2005b. *BiDil®* Package Insert. Lexington, MA: NitroMed.

NitroMed. 2005c. *Annual Report 2004*. Lexington, MA: NitroMed.

NitroMed. 2005d. CFDA Advisory Committee recommends approval for NitroMed's BiDil® to treat black patients with heart failure. *NitroMed® Key News*, July 16.

NitroMed. 2005e. *NitroMed Analyst Day: BiDil Launch Overview*. [Online]. Available at: http://www.lexisnexis.com [accessed: March 9, 2008].

NitroMed. 2006a. Risk to African Americans. [Online]. Retrieved from: http://www.hearthealthheritage.com/risk.asp [accessed: March 24, 2008].

NitroMed. 2006b. Advances in heart failure treatment in African Americans. [Online]. Retrieved from: http://www.hearthealthheritage.com/treating_advances.asp [accessed: March 24, 2008].

NitroMed. 2007a. BiDil®. [Online]. Retrieved from: http://www.nitromed.com/bidil/bidil.asp [accessed: March 23, 2008].

NitroMed. 2007b. BiDil® A-HeFT Trial. [Online]. Retrieved from: http://www.nitromed.com/bidil/aheft.asp [accessed: March 23, 2008].

NitroMed. 2007c. Genomic analysis. [Online]. Retrieved from: http://www.nitromed.com/bidil/genomic.asp [accessed: March 23, 2008].

NitroMed. 2007d. Common questions. [Online]. Available at: http://www.bidil.com/pnt/questions.php [accessed: February 28, 2008].

NitroMed. 2007e. Programs. [Online]. Retrieved from: http://www.bidil.com/pnt/programs.php [accessed: February 28, 2008].

NitroMed. 2008a. NitroMed reports on BiDil XR(TM) progress following FDA meeting, announces restructuring and suspension of BiDil® sales force, and retains investment bank to advise on strategic options. *NitroMed® Key News*, January 15. [Online]. Available at: http://investors.nitromed.com/phoenix.zhtml?c=130535&p=irol-newsArticle&ID=1096799&highlight, [accessed: September 2, 2008].

NitroMed. 2008b. NitroMed reports financial results for fourth quarter and full year 2007. *NitroMed® Key News*, February 14. [Online]. Available at: http://phx.corporate-ir.net/phoenix.zhtml?c=130535&p=irol-newsArticle&ID=1108225&highlight [accessed: September 2, 2008].

NitroMed. 2009. NitroMed announces agreement to be acquired by Deerfield Management; terminates agreements with Archemix Corp. and JHP Pharmaceuticals, LLC. *NitroMed® Key News*, January 27. [Online].

Available at: http://phx.corporate-ir.net/phoenix.zhtml?c=130535&p=irol-newsArticle&ID=1249340&highlight= [accessed: May 20, 2009].

NitroMed. n.d.a. *Heart Failure Backgrounder.* Lexington, MA: NitroMed.

NitroMed. n.d.b. *Following the Trail of Evidence: The BiDil® Story.* Lexington, MA: NitroMed.

Novas, C. 2009. Orphan drugs, patient activism and contemporary healthcare. *Quaderni*, 68, 13–23.

Obasogie, O.K. 2009. *Playing the Gene Card? A Report on Race and Human Biotechnology.* Oakland, CA: Center for Genetics and Society.

Office of Management and Budget (OMB). 1997. *Revisions to the Standards for the Classification of Federal Data on Race and Ethnicity.* [Online]. Available at: http://www.whitehouse.gov/omb/fedreg_1997standards [accessed: September 24, 2012].

Olopade, O.I., Fackenthal, J.D., Dunston, G., Tainsky, M.A., Collins, F. and Whitfield-Broome, C. 2003. Breast cancer genetics in African Americans. *Cancer*, 97(S1), 236–45.

O'Malley, P. 1992. Risk, power, and crime prevention. *Economy and Society*, 21(3), 252–75.

O'Malley, P. 1999. Social Justice after the "death of the social." *Social Justice*, 26(2), 92–100.

Omi, M. and Winant, H. 1994. *Racial Formation in the United States: From the 1960s to the 1990s.* 2nd Edition. New York: Routledge.

Ong, A. 2006. Mutations in citizenship. *Theory, Culture & Society*, 23(2–3), 499–505.

Organization for Economic Cooperation and Development (OECD). 2006. *The Bioeconomy to 2030: Designing a Policy Agenda.* Paris: OECD.

Osborne, T. and Rose, N. 1999. Governing cities: notes on the spatialization of virtue. *Environment and Planning D: Society and Space*, 17(6), 737–60.

Ossorio, P. and Duster, T. 2005. Race and genetics: controversies in biomedical, behavioral, and forensic sciences. *American Psychologist*, 60(1), 115–28.

Perez, L.N. 2005. Testimony, in *Cardiovascular and Renal Drugs Advisory Committee.* Vol. 2. Center for Drug Evaluation and Research, US Food and Drug Administration. Washington, DC: US Department of Health and Human Services, 255–9.

Petersen, A.R. and Lupton, D. 1996. *The New Public Health: Health and Self in the Age of Risk.* London: Sage.

Petryna, A. 2002. *Life Exposed: Biological Citizens After Chernobyl.* Princeton, NJ: Princeton University Press.

Petryna, A. 2006. The pharmaceutical nexus, in *Global Pharmaceuticals: Ethics, Markets, Practices*, edited by A. Petryna, A. Lakoff and A. Kleinman. Durham, NC: Duke University Press, 1–32.

Pollock, A. 2012. *Medicating Race: Heart Disease and Durable Preoccupations with Difference*. Durham, NC: Duke University Press.

PR Newswire. 1996. Medco Research files NDA for BiDil®. [Online]. Available at: http://www.thefreelibrary.com/MEDCO+RESEARCH+FILES+NDA+FOR+BIDIL(R)-a018449474 [accessed: May 30, 2013].

PR Newswire. 1999. NitroMed acquires BiDil™ New Drug Application for treatment of congestive heart failure. [Online]. Available at: http://www.thefreelibrary.com/NitroMed+Acquires+BiDil(TM)+New+Drug+Application+for+Treatment+Of [accessed: May 30, 2013].

PR Newswire. 2001. NitroMed initiates confirmatory BiDil® trial in African American heart failure patients. [Online]. Available at: http://www.prnewswire.com/news-releases/nitromed-initiates-confirmatory-bidil-r-trial-in-african-american-heart-failure-patients-71710052.html [accessed: July 12, 2008].

PR Newswire. 2007. Civil rights and medical leaders call for social justice in health care. [Online]. Available at: http://www.nmqf.org/press/Press%20Release_9-26-07_final-2.pdf [accessed: July 30, 2008].

Proctor, R.N. 1995. The destruction of "lives not worth living," in *Deviant Bodies: Critical Perspectives on Difference in Science and Popular Culture*, edited by J. Terry and J. Urla. Bloomington: Indiana University Press, 170–96.

Puckrein, G.A. 2005. Testimony, in *Cardiovascular and Renal Drugs Advisory Committee*. Vol. 2. Center for Drug Evaluation and Research, US Food and Drug Administration. Washington, DC: US Department of Health and Human Services, 210–14.

Rabinow, P. 1989. *French Modern: The Norms and Forms of the Social Environment*. Cambridge, MA: MIT Press.

Rabinow, P. 1996. *Essays on the Anthropology of Reason*. Princeton, NJ: Princeton University Press.

Rabinow, P. 1998. French enlightenment: truth and life. *Economy and Society*, 27(2–3), 193–201.

Rabinow, P. 1999. *French DNA: Trouble in Purgatory*. Chicago: University of Chicago Press.

Rabinow, P. 2005. Artificiality and enlightenment: from sociobiology to biosociality, in *Anthropologies of Modernity: Foucault, Governmentality, and Life Politics*, edited by J.X. Inda. Malden, MA: Wiley-Blackwell, 181–93.

Rabinow, P. and Rose, N. 2003. Introduction: Foucault today, in *The Essential Foucault*, edited by P. Rabinow and N. Rose. New York: New Press, vii–xxxv.

Rabinow, P. and Rose, N. 2006. Biopower today. *Biosocieties*, 1(2), 195–217.

Rapp, R., Taussig, K.S. and Heath, D. n.d. Standing on the biological horizon. Unpublished manuscript, Department of Anthropology, New York University.

Reardon, J. 2005. *Race to the Finish: Identity and Governance in an Age of Genomics.* Princeton, NJ: Princeton University Press.

Rector, R. 2004. *Welfare Reform: Progress, Pitfalls, and Potential.* [Online]. Available at: http://www.heritage.org/research/reports/2004/02/welfare-reform-progress-pitfalls-and-potential [accessed: November 11, 2013].

Redfield, P. 2005. Doctors, borders, and life in crisis. *Cultural Anthropology*, 20(3), 328–61.

Reid, J. 2006. Life struggles: war, discipline, and biopolitics in the thought of Michel Foucault. *Social Text*, 42(1), 127–52.

Reuters Health Medical News. 1997. FDA panel votes against Medco CHF combination drug. [Online]. Available at: http://www.lexisnexis.com [accessed: 22 July, 2008].

Reverby, S.M. 2009. *Examining Tuskegee: The Infamous Syphilis Study and Its Legacy.* Chapel Hill: University of North Carolina Press.

Risch, N.J. 2000. Searching for genetic determinants in the new millennium. *Nature*, 405, 847–56.

Risch, N., Burchard, E., Ziv, E. and Tang, H. 2002. Categorization of humans in biomedical research: genes, race, and disease. *Genome Biology*, 3(7), 1–12.

Roberts, D. 1997. *Killing the Black Body: Race, Reproduction, and the Meaning of Liberty.* New York: Pantheon Books.

Roberts, D. 2011a. What's wrong with race-based medicine? Genes, drugs, and health disparities. *Minnesota Journal of Law, Science & Technology*, 12(1), 1–21.

Roberts, D. 2011b. *Fatal Invention: How Science, Politics, and Big Business Re-Create Race in the Twenty-First Century.* New York: New Press.

Root, M. 2003. The use of race in medicine as a proxy for genetic differences. *Philosophy of Science*, 70(5), 1173–83.

Rosamond, W., Flegal, K., Friday, G., Furie, K., Go, A., Greenlund, K. et al. 2007. Heart disease and stroke statistics—2007 update: a report from the American Heart Association Statistics Committee and Stroke Statistics Subcommittee. *Circulation*, 115, e69–e171.

Rose, N. 1996a. The death of the social? Re-figuring the territory of government. *Economy and Society*, 25(3), 327–56.

Rose, N. 1996b. Governing "advanced" liberal democracies, in *Foucault and Political Reason: Liberalism, Neo-Liberalism, and Rationalities of Government*, edited by A. Barry, T. Osborne and N. Rose. Chicago: University of Chicago Press, 37–64.

Rose, N. 1996c. Psychiatry as a political science: advanced liberalism and the administration of risk. *History of the Human Sciences*, 9(2), 1–23.

Rose, N. 1999. *Powers of Freedom: Reframing Political Thought.* Cambridge, UK: Cambridge University Press.

Rose, N. 2000a. Governing liberty, in *Governing Modern Societies*, edited by R.V. Ericson and N. Stehr. Toronto: University of Toronto Press, 141–76.

Rose, N. 2000b. Government and control. *British Journal of Criminology*, 40(2), 321–39.

Rose, N. 2001. The politics of life itself. *Theory, Culture, & Society*, 18(6), 1–30.

Rose, N. 2006. Introduction to the discussion of race and ethnicity in nature genetics. *Biosocieties*, 1(3), 307–11.

Rose, N. 2007. *The Politics of Life Itself: Biomedicine, Power, and Subjectivity in the Twenty-First Century*. Princeton, NJ: Princeton University Press.

Rose, N. and Novas, C. 2005. Biological citizenship, in *Global Assemblages: Technology, Politics, and Ethics as Anthropological Problems*, edited by A. Ong and S.J. Collier. Malden, MA: Wiley-Blackwell, 439–63.

Rosenberg, N.A., Pritchard, J.K., Weber, J.L., Cann, H.M., Kidd, K.K., Zhivotovsky, L.A. et al. 2002. Genetic structure of human populations. *Science*, 298, 2381–5.

Rotman, D. 2005. Race and medicine. *Technology Review*, April, 60–65.

Rotter, J.I., Taylor, K.D., Guo, X., Goodarzi, M.O., Chen, Y.I., Raffel, L. et al. 2012. Methods of diagnosing insulin resistance and sensitivity. US Patent 20120088245, filed April 12.

Rusert, B.M. and Royal, C.D.M. 2011. Grassroots marketing in a global era: more lessons from BiDil. *Journal of Law, Medicine & Ethics*, 39(1), 79–90.

Sankar, P. 2006. Hasty generalisation and exaggerated certainties: reporting genetic findings in health disparities research. *New Genetics and Society*, 25(3), 249–64.

Sankar, P., Cho, M.K., Condit, C.M., Hunt, L.M., Koenig, B., Marshall, P. et al. 2004. Genetic research and health disparities. *Journal of the American Medical Association*, 291(24), 2985–9.

Sankar, P. and Kahn, J. 2005. BiDil: race medicine or race marketing? *Health Affairs*, 24, 455–63.

Saul, S. 2005a. US to review drug intended for just one race. *The New York Times*, June 13. [Online]. Available at: http://query.nytimes.com/gst/fullpage.html?res=9B05E0D61E38F930A25755C0A9639C8B63 [accessed: October 9, 2013].

Saul, S. 2005b. Maker of heart drug intended for blacks bases price on patients' wealth. *The New York Times*, July 8. [Online]. Available at: http://www.nytimes.com/2005/07/08/business/08hdrug.html?pagewanted=all&_r=0 [accessed: October 10, 2013].

Saunders, E., Smith, W.B., DeSalvo, K.B. and Sullivan, W.A. 2007. The efficacy and tolerability of nebivolol in hypertensive African American patients. *Journal of Clinical Hypertension*, 9(1), 866–75.

Savard, J. 2013. Personalized medicine: a critique of the future of health care. *Bioethical Inquiry*, 10(2), 197–203.

Schmitt, C. 1985. *Political Theology: Four Chapters on the Concept of Sovereignty*. Cambridge, MA: MIT Press.

Schneiderman, L. and Schneiderman, E. 2001. Proposed laws don't address actual issues. *Los Angeles Times*, July 8, M2.

Schram, S.F. 2000. *After Welfare: The Culture of Postindustrial Social Policy*. New York: New York University Press.

Seccombe, K. and Hoffman, K.A. 2007. *Just Don't Get Sick: Access to Health Care in the Aftermath of Welfare Reform*. New Brunswick, NJ: Rutgers University Press.

Séguin, B., Hardy, B., Singer, P.A. and Daar, A.S. 2008. BiDil: recontextualizing the race debate. *Pharmacogenomics Journal*, 8(3), 169–73.

Sehgal, A.R. 2004. Overlap between whites and blacks in response to antihypertensive drugs. *Hypertension: Journal of the American Heart Association*, 43(3), 566–72.

Shaefer, H.L. and Edin, K. 2012. *Extreme Poverty in the United States, 1996 to 2011*. Ann Arbor, MI: National Poverty Center.

Shields, A.E., Fortun, M., Hammonds, E.M., King, P.A., Lerman, C., Rapp, R. et al. 2005. The use of race variables in genetic studies of complex traits and the goal of reducing health disparities: a transdisciplinary perspective. *American Psychologist*, 60(1), 77–103.

Smedley, B.D., Stith, A.Y. and Nelson, A.R. 2003. *Unequal Treatment: Confronting Racial and Ethnic Disparities in Health Care*. Washington, DC: National Academies Press.

Stepan, N. 1982. *The Idea of Race in Science: Great Britain 1800–1960*. Hamden, CT: Archon Books.

Stoddard, L. 1921. *The Rising Tide of Color Against White World-Supremacy*. New York: Scribner's.

Stoler, A.L. 1995. *Race and the Education of Desire: Foucault's* History of Sexuality *and the Colonial Order of Things*. Durham, NC: Duke University Press.

Sunder Rajan, K. 2006. *Biocapital: The Constitution of Postgenomic Life*. Durham, NC: Duke University Press.

Sunder Rajan, K. 2007. Experimental values: Indian clinical trials and surplus health. *New Left Review*, 45, 67–88.

Sunder Rajan, K. 2012a. Introduction: the capitalization of life and the liveliness of capital, in *Lively Capital: Biotechnologies, Ethics, and Governance in Global Markets*, edited by K. Sunder Rajan. Durham, NC: Duke University Press, 2–41.

Sunder Rajan, K. 2012b. Pharmaceutical crises and questions of value: terrains and logics of global therapeutic politics. *South Atlantic Quarterly*, 111(2), 321–46.

Tate, S.K. and Goldstein, D.B. 2004. Will tomorrow's medicines work for everyone? *Nature Genetics*, 36(11), S34–S42.

Tavernise, S. and Gebeloff, R. 2013. Millions of poor are left uncovered by health law. *The New York Times*, October 2. [Online]. Available at: http://www.

nytimes.com/2013/10/03/health/millions-of-poor-are-left-uncovered-by-health-law.html?_r=0 [accessed: November 25, 2013].

Taylor, A.L., Ziesche, S., Yancy, C., Carson, P., D'Agostino, R., Ferdinand, K. et al. 2004. Combination of isosorbide dinitrate and hydralazine in blacks with heart failure. *New England Journal of Medicine*, 351(2), 2049–57.

Taylor, Malcolm P. n.d. *Frequently Asked Questions About the A-HeFT Trial: Background for ABC Members*. Washington, DC: Association of Black Cardiologists.

Temple, R. and Stockbridge, N.L. 2007. BiDil for heart failure in black patients: the US Food and Drug Administration perspective. *Annals of Internal Medicine*, 146(1), 57–62.

Thomaselli, R. 2005. Heart drug for blacks raises hackles on ethics. *Advertising Age*, January 24. [Online]. Available at: http://adage.com/article/news/heart-drug-blacks-raises-hackles-ethics/101839 [accessed: October 10, 2013].

Ticktin, M.I. 2011. *Casualties of Care: Immigration and the Politics of Humanitarianism in France*. Berkeley: University of California Press.

Trisi, D. and Pavetti, L. 2012. *TANF Weakening as a Safety Net for Poor Families*. Washington, DC: Center on Budget and Policy Priorities.

Trock, B.J. 1996. Breast cancer in African American women: epidemiology and tumor biology. *Breast Cancer Research and Treatment*, 40(1), 11–24.

Tutton, R. 2012. *Patient Advocacy, Biosociality and Other Identity Practices*, ESRC Genomics Network Annual Conference, London, UK, April 23, 2012.

Urban, T.J. 2010. Race, ethnicity, ancestry, and pharmacogenetics. *Mount Sinai Journal of Medicine*, 77, 133–9.

US Census Bureau. 2005. *Directive No. 15: Race and Ethnic Standards for Federal Statistics and Administrative Reporting*. [Online]. Available at: http://wonder.cdc.gov/wonder/help/populations/bridged-race/Directive15.html [accessed: September 24, 2012].

US Department of Health and Human Services (US DHHS). 1991. *Healthy People 2000: National Health Promotion and Disease Prevention Objectives*. Washington, DC: US Department of Health and Human Services.

US Department of Health and Human Services (US DHHS). 2000a. *Healthy People 2010: Understanding and Improving Health*. Washington, DC: US Department of Health and Human Services.

US Department of Health and Human Services (US DHHS). 2000b. Change in TANF caseloads since enactment of new welfare law. [Online]. Retrieved from: http://www.acf.hhs.gov/news/stats/aug-dec.htm [accessed: June 30, 2004].

US Department of Health and Human Services (US DHHS). 2013. TANF: total number of recipients. [Online]. Available at: https://www.acf.hhs.gov/sites/default/files/main/2013_recipient_tan.pdf [accessed: December 11, 2013].

US Food and Drug Administration (US FDA). 1997a. *Eightieth Meeting of the Cardiovascular and Renal Drugs Advisory Committee*, Center for Drug Evaluation and Research, US Food and Drug Administration. Washington, DC: US Department of Health and Human Services.

US Food and Drug Administration (US FDA). 1997b. *Cardiovascular and Renal Drugs Advisory Committee 80th Meeting: Minutes*, Center for Drug Evaluation and Research, US Food and Drug Administration. Washington, DC: US Department of Health and Human Services.

US Food and Drug Administration (US FDA). 2005a. *Cardiovascular and Renal Drugs Advisory Committee*. Vol. 2. Center for Drug Evaluation and Research, US Food and Drug Administration. Washington, DC: US Department of Health and Human Services.

US Food and Drug Administration (US FDA). 2005b. FDA approves BiDil heart failure drug for black patients. [Online]. Available at: http://www.fda.gov/NewsEvents/Newsroom/PressAnnouncements/2005/ucm108445.htm [accessed: April 27, 2011].

US Food and Drug Administration (US FDA). 2005c. *Guidance for Industry Collection of Race and Ethnicity Data in Clinical Trials*. Rockville, MD: US Food and Drug Administration.

Veiga, R.V. and Taylor, R.E. 1986. Beta blockers, hypertension, and blacks—is the answer really in? *Journal of the National Medical Association*, 78(9), 851–6.

Wacquant, L. 2010. Crafting the neoliberal state: workfare, prisonfare, and social insecurity. *Sociological Forum*, 25(2), 197–220.

Wailoo, K. 2001. *Dying in the City of Blues: Sickle Cell Anemia and the Politics of Race and Health*. Chapel Hill: University of North Carolina Press.

Wailoo, K. 2011. *How Cancer Crossed the Color Line*. Oxford, UK: Oxford University Press.

Wailoo, K., Nelson, A. and Lee, C. (eds). 2012. *Genetics and the Unsettled Past: The Collision of DNA, Race, and History*. New Brunswick, NJ: Rutgers University Press.

Wailoo, K. and Pemberton, S. 2006. *The Troubled Dream of Genetic Medicine: Ethnicity and Innovation in Tay-Sachs, Cystic Fibrosis, and Sickle Cell Disease*. Baltimore: Johns Hopkins University Press.

Waldby, C. 2000. *The Visible Human Project: Informatic Bodies and Posthuman Medicine*. New York: Routledge.

Waldby, C. 2002. Stem cells, tissue cultures, and the production of biovalue. *Health: An Interdisciplinary Journal for the Social Study of Health, Illness, and Medicine*, 6(3), 305–23.

Waldby, C. and Cooper, M. 2008. The biopolitics of reproduction: post-Fordist biotechnology and women's clinical labour. *Australian Feminist Studies*, 23(55), 57–73.

Washington, H.A. 2006. *Medical Apartheid: The Dark History of Medical Experimentation on Black Americans from Colonial Times to the Present.* New York: Harlem Moon.

Washington Legal Foundation. 2008. WLF petitions CMS to revise reimbursement policies for BiDil. Washington Legal Foundation press release, August 7. [Online]. Available at: http://www.wlf.org/upload/080708rs.pdf [accessed: December 11, 2013].

Wehling, P. 2011. Biology, citizenship and the government of biomedicine: exploring the concept of biological citizenship, in *Governmentality: Current Issues and Future Challenges*, edited by U. Bröckling, S. Krasmann and T. Lemke. New York: Routledge, 225–46.

Weir, L. 2006. *Pregnancy, Risk, and Biopolitics: On the Threshold of the Living Subject.* New York: Routledge.

Weir, M.R., Gray, J.M., Paster, R. and Saunders, E., for the Trandolapril Multicenter Study Group. 1995. Differing mechanisms of action of angiotensin-converting enzyme inhibition in black and white hypertensive patients. *Hypertension*, 26, 124–30.

Westphal, S.P. 2006. Heart medication for blacks faces uphill battle. *Wall Street Journal*, October 16. [Online]. Available at: http://www.post-gazette.com/pg/06289/730462-114.stm [accessed: September 2, 2008].

White House. 2012. *National Bioeconomy Blueprint.* Washington, DC: White House.

Whitmarsh, I. 2008. *Biomedical Ambiguity: Race, Asthma, and the Contested Meaning of Genetic Research in the Caribbean.* Ithaca, NY: Cornell University Press.

Whitmarsh, I. 2009. Medical schismogenics: compliance and "culture" in Caribbean biomedicine. *Anthropological Quarterly*, 82(2), 447–75.

Whitmarsh, I. and Jones, D.S. (eds). 2010. *What's the Use of Race? Modern Governance and the Biology of Difference.* Cambridge, MA: MIT Press.

Williams, D. and Collins, C. 2001. Racial residential segregation: a fundamental cause of racial disparities in health. *Public Health Reports*, 116, 404–16.

Williams, R.A. 2007. The Association of Black Cardiologists: a small-group success story, in *Eliminating Healthcare Disparities in America: Beyond the IOM Report*, edited by R.A. Williams. Totowa, NJ: Humana Press, 307–12.

Winstein, K.J. 2007. NAACP presses US on heart drug. *Wall Street Journal*, January 25. [Online]. Available at: http://online.wsj.com/news/articles/SB116969437637987200 [accessed: October 10, 2013].

Yancy, C. 2002. The role of race in heart failure therapy. *Current Cardiology Reports*, 4(3), 218–25.

Yancy, C. 2007. The Association of Black Cardiologists responds to "race in a bottle": a misguided passion. *Scientific American*, July 30. [Online]. Available at: http://www.scientificamerican.com/article.cfm?id=the-association-of-black-cardiologists-responds-to-article [accessed: June 4, 2008].

Ziesche, S., Cobb, F.R., Cohn, J.N., Johnson, G. and Tristani, F., for the V-HeFT VA Cooperative Studies Group. 1993. Hydralazine and isosorbide dinitrate combination improves exercise tolerance in heart failure: results from V-HeFT I and V-HeFT II. *Circulation*, 87(6), VI-56–VI-64.

Index

A-HeFT trial 32–3, 52–3, 62, 66, 80
Acs, G. 102
active patient-consumers 87–8, 105
African Americans
  BiDil and racial biosociality 46–55
  biochemical materialization of hope 51–5
  breast cancer 60–1
  failure of BiDil to reach 105–6
  geneticization of race 61–5
  healthcare, lack of access to 51
  heart failure among 1–2
  and hypertension 71
  as injured and suffering population 47–51
  insurance, health, lack of access to 104–5
  medical experimentation on 15–16
  neglect, biomedical 50–1
  as niche market for BiDil 81–4
  nitric oxide (NO), ability to produce 62
  not seen as active patient-consumers 87–8, 105
  purchasing power of 82
  sickle cell anemia (SCA) 17, 44–5, 46, 67–8
Agamben, Giorgio 9–11
Alcon 89–90
"Artificiality and Enlightenment: From Sociobiology to Biosociality" (Rabinow) 40
Ashkenazi Jewish population, USA 44, 45–6
Association of Black Cardiologists (ABC) 49, 50, 51, 55, 63–4, 69–70
autism 108–9

bare life 9–10
Bayh-Dole Act 1980 77
BiDil
  A-HeFT trial 32–3, 52–3, 62, 66, 80
  advocacy efforts in support of 53–4
  African Americans and racial biosociality 46–55
  birth and development of 24–7
  cost of as high 85
  criticisms of 65–8
  decision against approval 26–7
  effect of 23
  as enhancer of nitric oxide (NO) 62
  failure to reach African Americans 105–6
  first trials of 23–4
  geneticization of race through 58, 61–5
  health disparities, reduction of 80
  insurance coverage 85
  market failure of 84–8
  marketing of 26, 32, 83–4
  mistrust of race-specific drugs 85–6
  niche market for 81–4
  passing reference to race initially 23–4
  patent applications 26, 32, 80–1
  physician skepticism of 86–7
  race focus 27–33

as race-specific, approval of 33–7, 64–5
race used to salvage 75, 80–1
rights connected to 105
use for African Americans as problematic 2–3
V-HeFT I and II trials 24–32, 75
vital value, racial 80
biochemical materialization of hope 51–5
bioeconomy
birth and growth of 76–7
life as central locus of value 77–8
niche marketing 79
vital value 77–9
biological citizenship 41–3
biologization of race 3
biopolitics defined 6–7
biopower
defined 6
forms of 6–7
individual responsibility, move to emphasis on 11–12
life-affirming qualities 11–13
literature focused on 8–13
molar to molecular understanding of life 12–13
and racism 7–8
and sovereign power 9–10
underside of 7–8, 9–11
bioscience
capitalization of 13, 76–7
vital value 78
biosociality
African Americans 44–5, 46
and citizenship 40–3
groups 42–6, 51–5
Jewish (Ashkenazi) population, USA 44, 45–6
racial 43–6
African Americans and BiDil 46–55
socio-environmental influences 45–6
biovalue 78n4
breast cancer 60–1
Brown, Wendy 97–8
Bystolic 90

camp, the 9–10
cancer, breast 60–1
capitalization of racial life 4–5
African Americans as market for drug 75
of bioscience 13, 76–7
life as central locus of value 77–8
niche marketing 79
vital value 77–9
see also neoliberalization of life
CHOICES 55
Christensen, Donna 2, 36–7, 70, 71
citizenship
biological 41–3
and biosociality 40–3
legal recognition 39
and neoliberalism 96–7
and pharmaceuticals 39
as theme in book 4
and welfarism 95
classification systems
molar based 14
molecular understanding of race 16–17
racial and ethnic categories 30–1, 35
Cofield, Juan 49, 85
Cohn, Jay 23, 24, 25–6, 27, 31–2, 80
commercial exploitation of science. *see* capitalization of racial life
communities, biosocial 42–3
African Americans 44–5, 46
BiDil and African Americans 51–5
Jewish (Ashkenazi) population, USA 44, 45–6
Community HeartBEAT 55

concentration camps 10
Condit, Celeste 86
contracts of mutual responsibility 100
Coumadin 91–2
Crawford, Robert 103–4
Crestor 91–2
Curry, Charles 54

dependency on welfare programs 98–9
difference findings 60–1
discipline 6
discrimination, potential for 67
disparities in health
  BiDil and reduction of 80
  concern to reduce 29, 34–6
  geneticization of race 68, 69
  NitroMed 54n8
  political concern to reduce 29
  and race 72–3
  racial 3–4
  racial and ethnic categories 30–1
dosing of drugs 91–2
Duster, Troy 70–1

Ecks, Stefan 107
economic exploitation of science, *see* capitalization of racial life
endothelial nitric oxide synthase (NOS3) gene 62–3
enlightened geneticization of race 57–8, 69–74
environmental factors as ignored 108–9
epistemological climate
  BiDil as race-specific, approval of 33–6
Epstein, Steven 25n2, 60, 72
ethical beings 97
ethnic minorities
  categories 30–1, 35
  underepresentation of in clinical research 25n2, 29–30, 35
  see also African Americans
eugenics project of Nazi Germany 14–15
experimentation on African Americans 15–16

Fassin, Didier 56
Ferdinand, Keith 49, 63–4, 69
Food and Drug Administration (FDA) 64–5
Food and Drug Administration Modernization Act 1997 30
Forest Laboratories 90
Foucault, Michel 5–8
Frank, Danielle 86–7

Genetic Risk Assessment in Heart Failure (GRAHF) 62, 70
geneticization of race
  BiDil 61–5
  breast cancer 60–1
  in contemporary science 58–61
  criticisms of 57
    and BiDil 65–8
  difference findings 60–1
  disputed link between race and disease 66–7
  enlightened geneticization 57–8, 69–74
  health disparities 68, 69
  stigmatization and discrimination, potential for 67
  through BiDil 58
genetics
  appeal of for neoliberalism 107–8
  endothelial nitric oxide synthase (NOS3) gene 62–3
  mapping of the human genome 16
  metabolization of drugs 28–9
  molecular understanding of race 16–17
  population 58–60

social environment as ignored 108–9
genomics
and BiDil as race-specific, approval of 34
Germany, eugenics during the Nazi period 14–15
Giroux, Henry 103
Glivec 107
Goldstein, David 61
groups, biosocial 42–3
African Americans 44–5, 46
BiDil and African Americans 51–5
Jewish (Ashkenazi) population, USA 44, 45–6
Guidance for Industry: Collection of Race and Ethnicity Data in Clinical Trials 35

Hacking, Ian 40n1
Harvey, David 76, 97
health disparities
BiDil and reduction of 80
concern to reduce 29, 34–6
geneticization of race 68, 69
NitroMed 54n8
political concern to reduce 29
and race 72–3
racial 3–4
racial and ethnic categories 30–1
health/illness, citizenship and 39
healthcare
individual responsibility in 103–5
lack of access to 51
"Healthcare Quality in America: A 21st Century Civil Rights Priority" press conference 54–5
healthism 103–5
Healthy People 2000: National Health Promotion and Disease Prevention Objectives 29
Healthy People 2010 34–5
heart failure among African Americans 1–2
Hedgecoe, Adam 57
Heritage Foundation 101
History of Sexuality, The (Foucault) 5–7
Hoffman, Sharona 67
Holocaust, Jewish 14–15
homo sacer 9n2
Homo Sacer: Sovereign Power and Bare Life (Agamben) 9–11
Human Genome Project 16, 34
hypertension 71

individual responsibility
barriers to 101
and biosocial groups 42
emphasis on 11–12
in healthcare 93–4, 103–5
individual responsibility plans 100
neoliberalism 96–7
neoliberalization of life 93–4
insurance, health
coverage for BiDil 85
lack of access to 104–5
International HapMap Project 34
International Society on Hypertension in Blacks 54

Jewish (Ashkenazi) population, USA 44, 45–6
Jewish Holocaust 14–15

Kahn, Jonathan 27, 66, 88
Keita, Shomarka 2–3
Kittles, Rick 71–2

Lee, Debra 1–2
life, racial politics of 3–4, 13–18
Loberg, Michael 50, 80, 83
Loprest, P. 102

making up people 40n1

mapping of the human genome 16
marketing
  of BiDil 26, 32, 79, 81–4, 84n8, 87–8
  and race 82
Medco 26
metabolization of drugs and genetics 28–9, 61
minorities
  categories 30–1, 35
  underepresentation of in clinical research 25n2, 29–30, 35
  see also African Americans
mistrust of race-specific drugs 85–6
molar to molecular understanding of life 12–13
molecular understanding of race 16–17
Moussatos, Liana 83
Moynihan, Daniel Patrick 98
Murray, Charles A. 98

Nadesan, Majia Holmer 108
National Association for the Advancement of Coloured People (NAACP) 49, 50, 51, 55
National Human Genome Research Institute (NHGRI) 36
National Institutes of Health (NIH) Revitalization Act 1993 30
National Medical Association 54
National Minority Health Foundation 54
Nazi Germany 14–15
neglect, biomedical, of African Americans 50–1
neoliberalization of life
  appeal of genetic medicine 107–8
  failure of BiDil to reach African Americans 105–6
  individual responsibility for health 93–4, 103–5
  insurance, health, lack of access to 104–5
  patient assistance program of NitroMed 106–7, 107n5
  precarization of life 97–103
  racialized medicine generally 107–8
  rights connected to BiDil 105
  welfare system, criticisms and reform of 98–103
  welfarism, move from to neoliberalism 94–7
  see also capitalization of racial life
niche marketing of pharmaceuticals 79
  BiDil 81–4
Nissen, Steven 64–5
nitric oxide (NO) 62
NitroMed
  biochemical materialization of hope 52–3
  development of BiDil 32
  geneticization of African Americans 62–3
  health disparities, reduction of 54n8
  market failure of BiDil 84–5, 87–8
  market for BiDil 83–4, 84n8
  patient assistance program 106–7
  race as genetic category 69–70
  sale to Arbor Pharmaceuticals 84–5
  suffering of African Americans 47–8, 50
Novartis 107
Novas, Carlos 41, 42–3

O'Malley, Pat 97

patent protection
  applications for BiDil 26, 32, 80–1
  and race 88–9
Pavao, Mark 83
Perez, Lucille 54
Personal Responsibility and Work Opportunity Reconciliation Act 1996 (Welfare Act) 99
pharmaceuticals

and citizenship 39
differentiation of products, use of race in 89–90
niche marketing of 79
pharmacogenetics
discoveries made in 28–9
formation of field 27–8
Pharmacogenomics and Risk of Cardiovascular Disease (PARC) 34
Pharmacogenomics Research Network (PGRN) 34
physician skepticism of race-specific drugs 86–7
political climate
BiDil as race-specific, approval of 33–6
health disparities, concern to reduce 29, 34–6
politics
natural life, exclusion from 9–11
racial politics of life 13–18
vital, exclusionary types 15–16
Pollock, Anne 107n5
population genetics 58–60
poverty, link with welfare reforms 102–3
power of death 7
precarization of life 97–103
Puckrein, Gary 54
purchasing power of African Americans 82

Rabinow, Paul 11–13, 16, 40–1, 78
race
biologization of 3
and biosociality 43–6
African Americans and BiDil 46–55
categories 30–1, 35
continuing value of 88–92
differentiation of products, use of in 89–90
and disparities in health 3–4
disputed link with disease 66–7
dosing of drugs 91–2
as genetic category 69–70
harms from racialized medicine 17–18
and health disparities 72–3
historical instability of 65–6
and marketing 82
and metabolization of drugs 28–9, 61
molecular understanding of 16–17
and niche marketing 81–4
and patent protection 88–9
as social phenomenon 70–1
as used to salvage BiDil 75, 80–1
within-group variation 72
see also geneticization of race
"Racial Differences in Response to Therapy for Heart Failure: Analysis of the Vasodilator-Heart Failure Trials" (Carson) 31–2
racial politics of life 3–4, 13–18
racism and biopower 7–8
Ramey, Leland 48–9, 53
recombinant DNA technology (RDT) 77
responsibility, individual
barriers to 101
and biosocial groups 42
emphasis on 11–12
in healthcare 93–4, 103–5
individual responsibility plans 100
neoliberalism 96–7
neoliberalization of life 93–4
rights
connected to BiDil 105
and health/illness as theme in book 4

Risch, Neil 59–60
Roberts, Dorothy 65–6, 68, 91–2, 109
Rose, Nikolas 11–13, 17, 41, 42–3, 95
Rosenberg, Noah 58
rosuvastatin 91–2

Sabolinski, Michael 52
Sankar, Pamela 73
Saunders, Elijah 90
schizophrenia genetics 57
Shelton, Hilary 49
sickle cell anemia (SCA) 17, 44–5, 46, 67–8
Smith, Andrew J. 85
social insurance 94–5
Society Must Be Defended (Foucault) 7–8
socio-environmental influences
  and biosociality 45–6
  as ignored 108–9
  racial disparities in health 73–4
sovereign power and biopower 9–10
state of exception 10
stigmatization and discrimination, potential for 67
Stockbridge, N.L. 37
Stoddard, Lothrop 15
Strategic Research Plan and Budget to Reduce and Ultimately Eliminate Health Disparities (NIH 2002) 35
Sunder Rajan, Kaushik 78

Tate, Sarah 61
Tay-Sachs disease (TSD) 44
Taylor, Malcolm 51
Temple, R. 37
Temporary Assistance for Needy Families (TANF) 99–100
Thompson, Tommy G. 101
Travatan 89–90
Tuskegee Syphilis Study 15–16

V-HeFT I and II trials 24–6, 75
  race, re-analysis of data for 27–32
vasodilators, tests of 24–5
Vigilante 83–4
vital rights
  connected to BiDil 105
  and health/illness as theme in book 4
vital value, racial
  African Americans as market for drug 75
  BiDil 80
  capitalization of bioscience 76–7
  definition of vital value 77–9
  life as central locus of value 77–8

Waldby, Catherine 78n4
warfarin 91–2
Washington, Harriet 15
Weiss, Kenneth 71–2
welfare system
  abandonment of the poor 102–3
  criticisms of 98–9
  dependency on 98–9
  individual responsibility plans 100
  monitoring of subjects 100
  poverty, link with reforms 102–3
  reform of 99–103
welfarism, move from to neoliberalism 94–7
Wells, Dianna 48, 53
within-group variation 72
women, underepresentation of in clinical research 25n2, 29–30, 35
Woodard, Larry 84
Worcel, Manuel 52

Yancy, Clyde 63, 70

For Product Safety Concerns and Information please contact our EU representative GPSR@taylorandfrancis.com Taylor & Francis Verlag GmbH, Kaufingerstraße 24, 80331 München, Germany

Batch number: 10725973

Printed by Printforce, the Netherlands